DATE	ISSUED TO
NO 27 '96	Lisa Byrd
DE. 8 '97	Beverly Collins

THE FACTS
ABOUT
CHEMOTHERAPY

THE FACTS
ABOUT
CHEMOTHERAPY

A Guide for
Cancer Patients
and Their Families

Paul R. Reich, M.D.,
with Janice E. Metcalf, M.S.

Consumer Reports Books
A Division of Consumers Union
Mount Vernon, New York

To my brother, Martin L. Reich, M.D. (1939–87)

Copyright © 1991 by Paul R. Reich, M.D.
Published by Consumers Union of United States, Inc.,
Mount Vernon, New York 10553,
by arrangement with K. S. Giniger Co., Inc., New York.

Library of Congress Cataloging-in-Publication Data

Reich, Paul Richard.
The facts about chemotherapy : the essential guide for cancer patients and
their families / Paul R. Reich with Janice E. Metcalf and the
editors of Consumer Reports Books.
p. cm.
Includes bibliographical references and index.
ISBN 0-89043-206-6 (hc).—ISBN 0-89043-207-4 (pb)
1. Cancer—Chemotherapy—Popular works.   I. Metcalf, Janice E.
II. Consumer Reports Books.   III. Title.
RC271.C5R43   1991
616.99'4061—dc20   90-20256
                                         CIP

Design by GDS / Jeffrey L. Ward
First printing, March 1991
Manufactured in the United States of America

Contents

Preface

Chemotherapy has become a major treatment for cancer. Patients and families need a source of information about chemotherapy to supplement, but not replace, the information provided by the treating physician. Informed patients can anticipate some of the problems they will face, be prepared to ask relevant questions, and be better able to make decisions about their therapy. I hope that some patients will even find some of their fears and anxieties alleviated by this information.

In this book I explain what cancer chemotherapy is all about. I describe the various drugs available for the treatment of specific cancers and how they are administered, as well as their side effects and their benefits. I also discuss how to select a specialist in cancer therapy—an oncologist—and how to evaluate a treatment center. And, just as important, I examine the costs of chemotherapy and sources of financial aid.

Family and friends of cancer patients who read this book will find that they understand more fully what patients with cancer face. If they are close to the patient, they may be better able to help make decisions about therapy and reduce fears and anxieties.

Health professionals and others who work with cancer patients can use this book to better understand their role in the management of cancer patients. This understanding will help them work more effectively with patients, patients' physicians, and colleagues.

Translating twenty years of experience with thousands of cancer patients into a readable and usable book has been difficult—mostly because of the tremendous amount of information and research available about the subject. I therefore combined the most current medical literature with my own views and the views of my colleagues. No attempt is made, however, to make this book all-inclusive or to document the scientific validity of every statement I make. To do so would only make this book difficult to read and understand.

I discuss guidelines for selecting an oncologist and cancer treatment center in Chapter 1, along with information about the costs of chemotherapy and sources of financial aid. In Chapter 2 I discuss the basic principles and terminology involved in selecting, administering, and evaluating a chemotherapy treatment program, and I cover the history of chemotherapy. Chapter 3 describes how new drugs are developed and tested. Chapter 4 deals with interpretation of recovery rates and ways to control pain. Chapters 5 and 6 describe how chemotherapy is used to cure cancer, or, at least, improve the quality of life. Chapters 7 and 8 describe drug side effects and their treatment, and special procedures related to chemotherapy. Also included is a list of useful resources.

Many of my patients and colleagues, particularly the oncology nurses in the Hematology-Oncology Unit at Beth Israel Hospital in Boston, have helped immeasurably with the writing of this book. I used their experiences to decide which material to include and how extensively it should be covered. I am grateful for their assistance. They convinced me that just knowing the issues can be a great help to cancer patients, who are about to undergo one of the most difficult trials of their lives.

Acknowledgments

Without the patience of my wife, Dianne, and my daughters, Sarah and Gwyn, this book would not have been written. I thank them for the time that should have been theirs, but was otherwise devoted to this book. My coauthor, Janice Metcalf, provided invaluable assistance in rewriting and editing this manuscript. Her insights and expertise are gratefully appreciated. Also, I would like to express my gratitude to my copublisher, Ken Giniger, who encouraged and helped me, in part, because of the tragic loss of his wife to cancer.

CHAPTER 1

Dealing with Cancer

Cancer in the United States Today

Cancer is a major killer of Americans, and it appears to be increasing as a cause of death. Each year, the American Cancer Society publishes the pamphlet *Cancer Facts and Figures,* which summarizes the state of cancer diagnosis and therapy in the United States. The statistics in the 1989 edition give a realistic view of the number of patients and families affected by this disease.

From 1930 to 1986, the number of cancer deaths in the general population increased by 20 percent. The American Cancer Society estimates that, in the 1980s, 9 million people developed some form of cancer and 4.5 million people died from the disease. An estimated 15 million Americans were under medical care for cancer during this decade. In 1989 alone, approximately 1 million people were diagnosed with cancer, and about 0.5 million died from the disease in that one year. Most alarming is the rise in the number of cases of lung cancer and the increased number of deaths attributed to this malignancy. Except for lung cancer, the death rates

for other common cancers, such as breast, colon, uterine, and prostate, have either remained the same or decreased slightly. Since
cancer will strike at some time in three out of four families, and
ultimately cause one of every five deaths in the United States, information about the prevention, early diagnosis, and treatment of
cancer has become increasingly important.

Despite intensive research efforts, we still do not know the cause
of most cancers. Certainly family history plays an important role,
especially in breast and colon cancer; the risk of developing these
diseases is increased if close family members have already been
diagnosed with the disease. Lung cancer, bladder cancer, and cancer of the mouth and throat are strongly associated with cigarette
smoking. Uterine cervical cancer rates are highest among women
who have engaged in sex at an early age and with multiple partners.
And as many of us know, excessive exposure to sunlight carries an
increased risk of developing skin cancer. Some cancers are almost
certainly caused by occupational and environmental factors, such
as exposure to cancer-causing materials like asbestos, vinyl chloride,
or benzene.

For 1989 the American Cancer Society estimated that most new
cancers in men were lung, prostate, colon, oral, and skin. The most
common new cancers in women were breast, colon, lung, uterine,
and skin. Unfortunately the most common cancers are not those
most likely to be cured by modern-day surgery, chemotherapy, or
radiation treatments.

Recent Developments

Despite the enormous and expensive efforts of the National Cancer Institute (an agency of the federal government) and the American Cancer Society (the largest source of private research funds
in the United States), cancer survival rates have improved little if
at all. Major advances in the treatment of leukemias, lymphomas,
and rare tumors of the reproductive system have led to improved
survival rates in those conditions, but these malignancies are relatively rare and account for only a small proportion of cancer
deaths. For example, the survival rates (cure) for childhood leu-

kemia have improved from approximately 20 percent about ten years ago to at least 60 percent with current therapy. Drug therapy for advanced cancer of the testicle has brought survival rates to 90 percent or more, when forty years ago the disease was almost uniformly fatal. Certain rare, fatal forms of lymphoma that were previously untreatable now can be controlled with drug therapy for many years without side effects. Research is continuing in the hope that equally successful therapies can be found to improve the survival rates for common cancers, such as lung, breast, colon, and prostate.

Two areas among the most active in the field of chemotherapy research are genetic engineering and bone marrow transplantation. Genetic engineering enables the manufacture of large quantities of naturally occurring substances that can be used as powerful drugs to combat cancer cells. For example, interferon, a protein produced by the body to fight off viral infections, turns out to have anticancer properties. When given in large doses to patients with some types of lymphomas and leukemia, the tumors shrink. Interferon is now being tested against advanced kidney tumors, for which there is currently no treatment, and against advanced melanoma, a skin tumor that is often fatal. Genetic engineering is producing large quantities of other naturally occurring substances as well, including: (1) tumor necrosis factor, which attacks tumors directly and destroys them (at least in the test tube); (2) interleukin-2, which activates the body's normal defenses against cancer cells; and (3) bone marrow growth regulators that prevent some of the side effects associated with cancer drug therapy. It is hoped that some of these substances will ultimately contribute to an increased survival rate for common tumors.

Genetic engineering also permits the production of monoclonal antibodies that recognize and destroy cancer cells, especially early in the course of the disease. These antibodies are now being tested for their ability to kill tumor cells while sparing normal cells. Although the results so far are not encouraging, efforts are continuing, since such an approach, if successful, may lead to therapy with fewer side effects than current treatments.

The second important research technique being used to improve cancer survival is bone marrow transplantation. Twenty years ago, it was discovered that patients with aplastic anemia or leukemia could be treated by a transplant of bone marrow from another individual with the same tissue type. Patients with aplastic anemia have an injured bone marrow that will not produce the blood cells that fight infection and bring oxygen to body tissues. Often there is no apparent cause for the condition. It is known, however, that aplastic anemia can be caused by drugs, such as the antibiotic chloramphenicol, or radiation, such as that produced in the Chernobyl nuclear reactor accident. Other recognizable causes include viruses, such as those that cause infectious hepatitis, and certain so-called autoimmune diseases in which the patient's body makes antibodies against its own bone marrow cells.

In leukemia, the patient's malignant cells destroy normal cells in the bone marrow. Drugs used to treat leukemia can completely kill the malignant cells, but then the marrow must be repopulated with transplanted normal bone marrow cells in order to function again. (In later chapters, I discuss situations in which bone marrow transplants are performed. The procedure itself is described in Chapter 8.) There are many problems with this new technique, but it is hoped that it can be adapted to treat common cancers such as breast, lung, and ovary, as well as the lymphomas and leukemias that are often treatable with these transplants.

Besides the massive and expensive research projects being pursued with genetic engineering and marrow transplants, a unique cancer treatment is being evaluated on a small scale. Investigators know of substances that interfere with the normal metabolism of cells and cause the buildup of toxic products. Although these products destroy both normal and cancer cells, cancer cells are especially vulnerable. The drug 2-chlorodeoxyadenosine (2-CDA) is an example. It was specifically developed to interfere with metabolism of white blood cells, the cells that become malignant in leukemia. Toxic substances released during the process are harmful to all white cells, but particularly to malignant ones. As the toxic substances accumulate, they preferentially destroy the malignant cells, which are more susceptible to their effects. The advantage of this drug is that it is cheap to produce and has few side effects. However, only one or two types of leukemia respond to the drug, and there is no current evidence that this drug or similar drugs will work in the more common cancers.

Cancer Detection and Prevention

It can never be overstated that early detection is the closest thing to prevention of cancer. Recognizing this, the American Cancer Society has published a list of warning signs in the hope that patients will see a doctor for early diagnosis and treatment before the cancer spreads. Early warning signs include

- a persistent cough or a cough that produces blood
- bleeding from the rectum or a change in normal bowel habits, frequently manifested as black stools
- breast lump or fluid discharge from the nipple
- vaginal bleeding between normal menstrual periods or after menopause
- sores on the mouth or lips that do not heal
- in elderly men, difficulty urinating or blood in the urine
- difficulty swallowing
- skin ulcers that do not heal; or skin eruptions that change in size or color, bleed, discharge fluid, or become painful
- in children, frequent infections or bleeding from the nose or other sites may be early signs of leukemia.

As with most diseases, it is far more beneficial to prevent cancer than to treat it, in terms of both human suffering and dollars spent. The American Cancer Society recommends that everyone stop smoking or chewing tobacco. There is also evidence that inhaling the smoke of others' cigarettes—secondhand smoke—can increase your risk of lung cancer. These risks can be reduced by avoiding areas where smoking is permitted.

If you indeed smoke or chew tobacco, you should know that high alcohol consumption is associated with mouth and throat cancer, especially when combined with use of tobacco.

No matter what type of work you do, be aware of any exposure to cancer-causing chemicals such as asbestos, nickel, cadmium, benzene, or vinyl chloride in your workplace. And write to your congressional representatives to show your support of clean air measures and environmental laws to clean up and prevent pollution, which has already been linked to lung cancer.

Even measures as simple as avoiding excessive exposure to sunlight and radiation, such as radon or unnecessary medical and dental X rays, can help reduce your chances of getting cancer.

The role of nutrition and diet in preventing cancer is a matter of debate. No cause-and-effect relationship has been conclusively demonstrated between diet and the risk of developing cancer. The American Cancer Society does, however, recommend some very basic points, such as controlling your weight, reducing your alcohol consumption, cutting down on fats, and avoiding smoked and nitrite-cured foods, such as bacon or smoked sausages. They also advise people to eat more foods that are high in fiber, including foods containing vitamins A and C—for example, carrots, spinach, peaches, and apricots for vitamin A and citrus fruits for vitamin C.

Examinations that will detect early cancers are important preventive measures. Consult your physician for further information about these procedures. Here are some examples.

- for women: mammograms and breast self-examination for breast cancer, and Pap tests for uterine and cervical cancer
- for men: genital self-examinations
- for both: rectal examinations and tests for blood in the stool
- especially for individuals with a family history of colon cancer: proctoscopies and colonoscopies, which inspect the lining of the colon with a flexible tube inserted through the rectum (see Chapter 6).

Choosing Cancer Treatment

If you are a cancer patient, you are undoubtedly wondering what is ahead for you. You may be facing a great deal of uncertainty, and you may be asked to make some difficult decisions.

Biopsy and Surgery

Perhaps you noticed a lump, abnormal bleeding, or other symptoms of disease, for example, a cough. Perhaps an abnormality was found on an X ray or CAT scan, and your physician referred you to a surgeon for biopsy or removal of the tumor. A biopsy is generally performed to diagnose cancer, not to treat it, although the entire tumor may be removed during the biopsy. A small sample of the tumor is removed and prepared for viewing under a microscope. The presence of malignant cells in the biopsy specimen is an important way to diagnose cancer. Surgical treatment, on the other hand, generally removes the entire affected organ or part of an organ with the hope of curing the cancer.

Once the diagnosis of cancer is made and surgical treatment performed, the question of further therapy with radiation or chemotherapy is usually discussed with the surgeon in consultation with your physician. Often some discussion of these therapies takes place before the operation, but only after surgery can definite plans be made, since further treatment will depend on the type of cancer and if and how far it has spread. This information may not be available until after surgery and examination of the specimens removed.

Oncologist and Treatment Options

At this point, you may be referred to an oncologist, a physician who specializes in treating cancer. Most of your early appointments with the oncologist will be spent discussing options, such as drugs, immunotherapy, or hormone treatments. Sometimes more than one treatment option will be available to you. The oncologist will discuss potential benefits, side effects, and costs in great detail. (I

describe guidelines for choosing an oncologist later in this chapter.)
The type of oncologist you see will depend on your type of cancer:
hematologists treat lymphomas and leukemias, medical oncologists
treat all malignancies, gynecological oncologists treat only malignancies of the female reproductive organs, and pediatric oncologists treat only cancer in children. If there is reason to believe that
radiation therapy will be helpful, a third doctor will join the team,
a radiation therapist. A final treatment plan will result from these
discussions and, perhaps, a second opinion from another oncologist, who might be more experienced with treatment of your type
of cancer. When needed or requested by you or your family, a
second opinion is best arranged by the treating oncologist. In that
way, important information about you and your condition can be
efficiently transmitted to the oncologist who will give the second
opinion.

If any cancer cells remain after surgery, they *may* be destroyed
by the body's own defense mechanisms. However, after removal of
the tumor, the next step often is radiation treatment with high-
energy X rays to kill any cancer cells left behind after surgery in
or near the operative field. The use of radiation treatment depends
on the type of cancer and how far it has spread. Radiation is most
commonly recommended in patients where the cancer has spread
outside the organ that was initially removed. A patient with breast
cancer, for example, may require radiation treatment if the cancer
has spread beyond the affected breast or has spread locally to skin
or lymph nodes.

If radiation is part of your treatment plan, you will be sent to a
treatment center where physical examination by the radiation therapist combined with computer-assisted analysis of where the tumor
is located in your body will help determine your radiation treatment
plan. You will be told how many treatments you will need and the
approximate length of time you will be under the radiation-
producing machine. The times may vary as treatment proceeds.
Four or five days a week for anywhere from two to ten weeks, you
will report to the radiation treatment center, where you will be
positioned under a machine and a dose of radiation will be delivered, and then you will go home. Fatigue, nausea, and skin burns

are some of the usual side effects of radiation therapy. Your radiation therapist will describe these and other side effects prior to therapy, along with suggestions of how to alleviate them (see Chapter 8).

Chemotherapy as an Option

The newest therapy for cancer is chemotherapy. Chemotherapy is usually first mentioned just before or after a biopsy or surgery. Throughout this book, I focus on chemotherapy, but remember that it is only one of several treatment approaches available. The option of not doing any chemotherapy is always there if the cancer is one that responds poorly to available drugs or if the drugs used are particularly toxic. Sometimes it is better to maintain a good quality of life with pain medications and sedation than to try chemotherapy, especially if it is very likely to fail or to cause serious discomfort. Do not overlook this option in the rush to treat your cancer.

Chemotherapy is simply the use of chemicals (drugs) to treat cancer. Various drugs and combinations of drugs are used to (1) prevent cancer from coming back once the original tumor has been removed; (2) to cure patients whose disease has spread beyond the point where surgery is possible; or (3) to relieve symptoms caused by cancers that have spread to other parts of the body.

Chemotherapy can help prevent further spread of cancer if therapy begins when the disease is in its early stages. Lymph node cancer is one of the few conditions that can be cured by chemotherapy even after it begins to spread. Most chemotherapy, however, is administered to patients who suffer from cancers that cannot be totally removed by surgery but are causing illness or pain. Colon cancer that has spread to the liver, for example, causes pain in the abdomen. The chemotherapy will relieve the pain, but it will not cure the cancer.

There are many types of drugs to choose from. Hormones, such as estrogens, are used to treat certain patients with breast or prostate cancer. Antibodies, substances produced naturally by the body to defend itself against tumor cells, are duplicated in the laboratory and given to patients in the hope that they will kill cancer cells that cannot be destroyed with other drugs or radiation. Most recently, chemicals that modify the body's own defense mechanisms, so-called immunomodulators, have been used to treat cancer. The chemicals "turn on" the patient's own defense mechanisms to produce antibodies or other chemicals that enhance the performance of cells the body normally produces to destroy cancer cells. These drugs that enhance the body's defenses are just now being tested so their role in cancer chemotherapy can be determined.

If You Decide to Receive Chemotherapy

Once you decide to receive chemotherapy, you will be given an appointment to a treatment unit in a hospital, at a clinic, or in the oncologist's office. Nurses will be available to discuss your concerns and again review possible side effects. You may be asked to give oral or written permission for the physician to administer the chemotherapy. Only then will a tube be placed into your vein and the prescribed drugs administered. One treatment may last anywhere from five minutes to eight or more hours. After the drug dose is given, a nurse will check your vital signs (temperature, pulse rate, and blood pressure) and ask you if you have any discomfort. You will be given painkillers or other drugs and instructions for your care at home that night and during the next few days.

Since chemotherapy is often given in cycles, the treatment procedure will be repeated every two or three weeks for a period of months or even years. Your oncologist may need to change your chemotherapy drugs during the course of your treatments. Do not be alarmed if your oncologist suggests that different drugs are needed, either because the tumor has not responded or because further research has indicated that other drugs are more beneficial than those you received initially.

Especially after initial chemotherapy treatments, you may experience emotional problems. You may have trouble sleeping, or you may become depressed because of worry about the cancer and side effects of your treatments. You should discuss these problems with your oncologist, a nurse, or psychiatrists or social workers affiliated with the treatment unit. Your doctor may prescribe anti-anxiety or antidepression drugs to help with these symptoms, which are not caused by the drugs used to treat cancer.

You may anticipate side effects starting a few days before a scheduled treatment. You may feel anxious, nauseated, or may even vomit before actually receiving any drugs. Tell your doctor if you have these symptoms. Counseling and antianxiety medications can help reduce this anticipatory response as well.

How Cancer Develops

Cancer has many names—malignancy, tumor, neoplasm, carcinoma. Before being diagnosed as a tumor, a lump may be called a mass or a lesion. All these terms refer to a new growth of cells somewhere in the body. Cells are tiny structures, visible only under a microscope. They make up various body tissues which, in turn, make up organs and then systems. For example, bone cells, or osteocytes, make up bony tissue, individual bones, and then the entire skeletal system.

Each cell consists of cellular fluid, called cytoplasm, surrounding a central core, called a nucleus. The nucleus contains genetic material, or genes, that is responsible for controlling how a cell grows and reproduces. Cells divide by splitting the nucleus in a process called mitosis. Normally the cells divide in a controlled fashion, and the two "daughter cells" are genetically identical to the one "parent." In cancer, however, this process goes wild, leading to uncontrolled cell production (proliferation). The cancerous cells, also called malignant or neoplastic, grow so rapidly that they don't have time to mature properly, and they no longer resemble the original cell in terms of appearance or function. Therefore, they may look different when stained and examined under a microscope, and they may no longer make substances normally produced by previous cell generations.

The original location of a malignancy is called the primary site. If it spreads no farther, the malignant tumor is described as localized. Too often, however, cells travel from the primary site, setting up other locations, called secondary sites, for continued cell proliferation in other organs or throughout the body. This is known as systemic involvement. The spread of cancer to other locations is called metastasis (me-tas´ta-sis), and these secondary sites are then called metastases (me-tas´ta-ses).

The presence of cancer is often indicated by certain signs and symptoms in the patient. Signs are physical manifestations of the disease, such as altered blood levels or the finding of malignant cells, e.g., lumps somewhere in the body. These signs sometimes, but not always, cause symptoms, unusual body functions or feelings experienced by the patient. For example, patients with lung cancer may have severe chest pain, coughing, and difficulty breathing— symptoms of the cancer present in their lungs.

Some types of cancer, notably leukemias (cancers of the blood), are described as acute or chronic. An acute illness is one that comes on suddenly and progresses rapidly. A chronic illness develops slowly or remains unchanged over long periods of time. A low-grade malignancy is the term used for chronic conditions not likely to spread; a high-grade malignancy is acute and very likely to spread to other locations in the body.

Physicians often speak of cancer in terms of stages. Cancers are staged by oncologists based on physical examination, blood tests, and X rays. Early stages, usually called stages I and II, are characterized by no spread or local spread to nearby lymph nodes. In advanced stages, III and IV, cancer is found in areas distant from the original tumor and nearby lymph nodes, such as the lung, liver, or brain. Treatment is generally more effective in early stages rather than in later, advanced stages. Sometimes diagnosis is made of a precancerous condition, one which, left untreated, could develop into cancer.

The probable outcome of an individual's cancer is called the prognosis. A good prognosis means that there is a good chance that the disease can be cured or controlled. A poor prognosis means that there is little chance of destroying the cancer. The term *cure* has a different meaning with cancer than with other diseases. A cancer patient is considered cured if there is no evidence of disease for a specific period of time. Different time limits are set depending on the type of cancer. Breast cancer, for example, is not considered cured until the patient shows no evidence of disease for at least ten years.

Choosing an Oncologist

Most cancer patients are diagnosed by an internist or family physician, who then refers the patient to an oncologist, or cancer specialist. The following are important factors to consider when choosing an oncologist.

An Oncologist's Training

After graduating from medical school, physicians who plan on specializing in a particular field of medicine, such as internal medicine, take an internship of one year followed by a residency of at least two years in an approved hospital program. Following this training, they must pass an examination to become recognized as internists. An internist takes care of adult or adolescent medical problems but does not usually have special training in surgery, pediatrics (treating children), or obstetrics (treating pregnant women). To become a cancer specialist, or medical oncologist, an internist must complete three more years of training, called an oncology fellowship. The three years may include one year of clinical training and two years of research. During the research years, he or she will continue to take care of some cancer patients. This is done under the supervision of experienced oncologists, in a program approved for special training in cancer diagnosis and treatment, especially chemotherapy. The candidate oncologist must then pass a subspecialty examination in oncology to be recognized as an oncologist and cancer chemotherapist. After passing this examination, he or she is fully qualified to diagnose cancer, plan treatment, and administer chemotherapy.

Not all oncologists begin as internists. Many spend their residency training in pediatrics, for example, and then, after passing examinations in general pediatrics and receiving additional training in pediatric oncology, they qualify to treat children with cancer. Similarly, some surgeons and obstetrician-gynecologists obtain their credentials first in their specialty and then take further training to be recognized as oncologists. These particular doctors often practice surgical oncology. That is, they perform special cancer operations, but they do not administer anticancer drugs. Hematologists have subspecialty training in both hematology (diseases of the blood) and oncology, but some treat only blood-related cancers, such as leukemia and lymphomas. When choosing an oncologist, be aware that there are those who are recognized as such by their colleagues but who have not completed formal training or examinations in oncology. In the future, fewer and fewer physicians without formal training will deliver cancer chemotherapy. As the training becomes more defined and available, oncologists will be graduates of qualified programs and will have passed the special examinations in this field of medicine. Until then, it is in your interest to seek out a recognized oncologist, to ensure that you get the benefit of up-to-date research and treatment.

Particularly good oncology training programs are offered by specialized cancer centers throughout the country. Very often, family doctors will refer their patients to these centers or to one of their staff oncologists. If a physician either trained at, or was on the staff of, one of these centers, it is likely that he or she has adequate credentials. (See Appendix C for a selective list of these centers.)

Oncology Fellows

In many cancer centers and hospitals, cancer care is delivered by oncology fellows, who are in training and supervised to a varying degree by staff oncologists. Under supervision of an experienced staff oncologist, fellows become directly involved with cancer patients. Often they associate closely with patients and their families, participating in family events and visiting the patient at home. It is important, however, that fellows avoid becoming too close to their patients, and becoming depressed when and if some of their patients die.

Fellowship programs enable the physician in training to get experience with a wide range of patients with malignancies, including rare types. Fellows search the medical literature and consult with experts to learn about any new therapies that may help the patients under their care. In some cases, their interest leads to research projects that they undertake during the research years of their fellowship. Fellows can find themselves at the leading edge of research into cures for diseases they originally encountered while taking care of patients during these training years.

There are advantages and disadvantages to receiving care from these providers. Oncology fellows often have more time available to research the medical literature and to obtain multiple consultations from doctors specializing in one type of cancer. They are usually highly motivated and interested in their patients. On the other hand, they do not have the extensive experience of more senior oncologists. Most are very interested in patient-related problems, but some are thinking of careers in research and may not be particularly oriented to patient care. In any case, it is essential for patients to maintain some contact with the senior physicians supervising the oncology fellow, and if access is limited, it might be best to rely primarily on a full-time oncologist practicing outside the cancer center and use the senior oncologists and fellows at a center for consultation.

Board Certification

Most medical and some large public libraries have reference books that list the training and certifications of practicing specialists. These books include *Directory of Medical Specialists* (Marquis Who's Who, 200 East Ohio Street, Chicago, IL 60611) and *ABMS Compendium of Certified Medical Specialists* (American Board of Medical Specialties, Evanston, IL 60201). Physicians are listed by specialty and location—town or city. Each physician is described in terms of his or her training and certifications, such as medical oncology or hematology, certified by the American Board of Internal Medicine; or gynecologic oncology, certified by the American Board of Obstetrics and Gynecology. A physician board-certified in oncology is qualified by any standard to deliver cancer chemotherapy.

If your doctor is an internist, look first to see whether he or she has completed the necessary training and fellowships to qualify for examinations administered jointly by the American Board of Internal Medicine, American Medical Association, and the American College of Physicians for certification as a medical oncologist. If the doctor completed the training, he or she becomes board eligible, although this is not specifically stated in these reference books. Once the doctor passes the subspecialty examination, he or she is board certified and is listed as such in these directories.

Pediatricians are similarly examined by the American Board of Pediatrics in Pediatric Hematology–Oncology. Gynecologists wishing to be board-certified oncologists take examinations administered by the American Board of Obstetrics and Gynecology.

Other Considerations

Ask your oncologist if he or she has admitting privileges (the right to admit a patient) to a nearby hospital prepared to care for extremely ill patients, especially those with life-threatening infections and severe bleeding. University hospitals and cancer centers carefully supervise their staff and therefore offer an extra measure of assurance that a cancer patient is getting the best treatment. It is important to know the hospitals with which an oncologist is affiliated and also whether he or she holds a position in a university-affiliated medical school. This information should provide some assurance about the physician's training and ability to treat cancer patients. Hospital and medical school affiliations are also listed in the *Directory of Medical Specialists* and *ABMS Compendium of Certified Medical Specialists.*

Another important factor in selecting an oncologist is his or her reputation as a caring human being. The best source for this information, of course, is other patients or their families. Doctors who will make house calls when necessary, who participate in hospice or home health care programs, and who are available for telephone consultation are usually attuned to the emotional as well as physical needs of cancer patients. Patience, ability to listen to what the patient is saying, willingness to explain procedures and treatments, and availability for advice, especially when things are going badly, are all characteristics that patients should look for when choosing an oncologist.

The physician's philosophy about treating incurable cancer can be immensely important. There are oncologists who are very aggressive and keep advising chemotherapy even when the chances of returning the patient to a near normal life are small; other doctors will discuss withdrawing chemotherapy and looking after the patient's comfort during the last days or weeks of life. Of course, it is for you to decide, based on prognosis, to continue or discontinue treatment. Your own personality, needs, and wants should govern your choice of oncologist.

It's best to inform an oncologist about using life-support systems. For example, do you want to be resuscitated if your disease suddenly worsens to the point of heart or lung failure, especially if there is no hope of returning to a meaningful life? Other issues that should be discussed include: the use of mechanical breathing devices, requiring the insertion of a tube into the throat; feeding tubes passed into the stomach to maintain nutrition; and dialysis with artificial kidneys. Decisions do not need to be final; it is always possible to revise instructions to the physician as the disease and its treatment progress. Laws regarding this issue differ from state to state, and you should seek the advice of a lawyer as to how your wishes are to be carried out if you are too sick to communicate them.

Evaluating a Cancer Treatment Center

Physicians' offices, hospital outpatient units, cancer center clinics, and HMO (health maintenance organization) cancer units are all perfectly suitable for the administration of chemotherapy. The primary concerns are that the oncologist comes highly recommended and adequate physical facilities are available. Emergency equipment for severe drug reactions, adequate staff to treat and counsel patients, and access to acute hospital care for complications are essential no matter where the chemotherapy is actually administered. Since patients spend a lot of time in the facility while not feeling well, however, attractive surroundings, easy parking, reasonable waiting times, and a pleasant support staff are important pluses. It's a good idea to visit an inpatient or outpatient oncology unit before making a decision and starting treatment.

Cancer centers or special oncology units (see Appendix C) maintained by hospitals, HMOs, or other health care providers do have certain advantages. First, the staffs often include physicians who have interests in rare types of cancers, so consultation is readily available to patients with uncommon diseases. Second, these centers provide access to physicians who possess a knowledge of medical specialties necessary in managing the care of cancer patients and in controlling any complications caused by chemotherapy. These specialties include infectious disease, surgical and gynecological oncology, and blood banking. Finally, these centers' billing offices handle much of the paperwork necessary to settle financial matters, relieving patients and their families from the time-consuming task.

Beyond the doctor's credentials and center's facilities, there is a staff of other types of professionals trained to meet the specific needs of patients and their families. Specially trained oncology nurses add an immeasurable amount to the care of cancer patients and their families. These nurses take time to explain procedures, potential side effects, and ways to avoid discomfort or complications, and they make themselves readily available by phone to answer questions. They also counsel patients and families, refer patients to social workers and psychiatrists, and educate patients and families about nutritional matters. To alleviate the problem of scheduling treatments around job and family responsibilities, they often arrange for family members, friends, or social service organizations to provide support, transportation, and companionship before, during, and after treatment sessions. Well-staffed centers also include pharmacists specially trained to dispense cancer drugs, radiotherapists, social workers, and psychiatrists—also immediately available for consultation.

When appropriately organized and adequately supported, this

team approach to cancer and its therapy has important advantages, especially for those patients undergoing complex drug treatments and those who need assistance to solve economic or family problems. The only potential disadvantage is that some of these centers are staffed mainly by oncology fellows who, as previously described, are in training. Though fellows are usually highly motivated, they must be supervised by experienced senior oncologists. Therefore, it is necessary that the senior physician stays in regular contact with each patient to ensure the best of care.

You may want to consider inpatient cancer care. Many hospitals are quite successful at delivering such services. These include community hospitals and university-affiliated hospitals. Obviously, a well-trained staff is the most important consideration. These hospitals may or may not staff oncology fellows or interns and residents, but the Joint Commission on Accreditation of Health Care Organizations requires them to staff senior or attending oncologists and nurses trained to care for the special needs of cancer patients. As with cancer centers, their staffs must also include specialists in blood banking, infectious disease, neurology, and other fields of medicine that deal with complications of cancer and its therapy.

From the patient's point of view, other factors are, at least, of equal importance to staffing.

- Are the rooms clean and attractive?
- Is the hospital conveniently located, with easy parking?
- Is the support staff friendly and helpful?
- Are the visiting hours convenient?
- May a close family member stay with the patient, especially during acute illness?
- Is lodging available for family members who come from a distance and need to stay for short or extended periods of time?

With regard to lodging away from home, Ronald McDonald houses, supported by the fast-food chain, are available near some urban hospitals for families of children who have cancer. Bed-and-breakfast guest houses are another reasonably priced alternative to hotels or motels. Hospitals and treatment centers often have a list of available housing. Ask for information from your doctor, oncology nurses, hospital social service department, or the American Cancer Society.

Evaluating Cancer Treatment Plans

After choosing an oncologist and a place to administer chemotherapy, the next important step is developing the treatment plan itself. To begin with, you and your doctor should discuss whether or not chemotherapy is the best treatment, rather than radiotherapy, surgery, or no therapy at all. Again, although chemotherapy is the focus of this book, other treatment options may be preferable. Usually your doctor will present you with an outline of the proposed treatment plan, which will describe the drugs to be used, the dosing schedule, side effects, potential benefits, and whether or not you will need to be hospitalized. If you find that an experimental program is an option, you should discuss it in great detail, especially if you are choosing between receiving no treatment at all and trying a high-risk experimental program (see Chapter 3). Other items you and your doctor should discuss include: costs of treatment; equipment requirements, such as chemotherapy pumps; and the need for surgery or special devices. Your doctor should be honest, patient, and willing to repeat information so you and your family leave his or her office with a complete understanding of treatment plans and alternatives.

Of course, if a family member of yours is in need of treatment but is incapable of giving an informed consent to the treatment plan, you may want to consult a lawyer. If necessary, the courts can appoint guardians to listen, decide, and, if reasonable, formally give consent to the proposed plan.

You, of course, should get a second opinion, especially if you are considering two potentially equal treatment plans. Your family doctor, local medical association, or even health insurance companies themselves can recommend a physician who can give you a second opinion. Second opinions serve several purposes. First, they often confirm the findings and conclusions of the first oncologist, which will give you and your doctor added confidence in the proposed treatment and peace of mind. Second, overlooked findings or treatment alternatives may come to light. These suggestions may lead to therapies that improve your prognosis. Third, your insurance company may require a second opinion if expensive surgery or other treatments are proposed.

At this point, it is important that you be thoroughly informed why the proposed program is reasonable. If there is something you don't understand, you can sometimes clarify these issues by discussing them with your primary care doctor. Your oncologist must keep the referring primary physician informed of your progress or lack of progress with a given treatment program. If the program fails, your primary physician may take over your care.

Consider at this stage of treatment your family's needs, too. Interactions between you and your spouse, children, and other family members are very important. At this stage of planning, psychiatric counseling for you and your family can be very helpful, as can counseling by knowledgeable and caring members of the clergy. As patients embark on dangerous treatment with uncertain results, it becomes even more important to seek support available through psychology, their religious beliefs, or both. If you are concerned about who should be told what and when, keep in mind this general rule: before long, everyone in the immediate family should know about the cancer diagnosis. Therefore, it is best, in most cases, to tell your family yourself, as soon as possible, so they can begin to deal with the problem and sort out any questions, concerns, or emotions they will experience. Even children sense what is going on and imagine the situation is worse than it really is, and sometimes they blame themselves for a parent's or sibling's cancer. If you feel you and your family need professional assistance, contact any local cancer service agency or refer to the list in Appendix B. *Taking Time,* an excellent booklet that deals with support for people with cancer and the people who care about them, is available through the National Cancer Institute, Bethesda, Maryland 20205 as Publication No. 85-2059. How to tell friends, employers, and business associates is also covered in this publication.

Costs of Chemotherapy

The cost of cancer care is so high that only the richest of us could afford it without help from insurance or other sources. Not only is inpatient hospital care very costly, but the cost of physician's services; medical equipment; outpatient clinics with their teams of doctors, nurses, social workers, pharmacists, and others; and chemotherapy drugs themselves can rapidly use up savings and income.

You should feel free to discuss costs with your physicians, the hospital billing office, and other health care providers. Usually, insurance or public health programs, such as Medicare and state-run Medicaid, cover most medical costs of treating cancer. With the proliferation of health care plans today, however, it is important to check with the oncologist about his or her participation in these plans. Some health plans will not pay for or will only partially reimburse a patient for cancer care if the oncologist is not a member of the plan. Similarly, closed-panel plans, such as HMOs, may severely restrict your choice of an oncologist.

The first step is to minimize your out-of-pocket expenses—that is, costs that are not covered by insurance or other resources. Physicians fees not covered by standard insurance can be minimized for patients covered by special insurance plans that provide full coverage for serious illness. Many Blue Shield plans, for example, give full coverage to cancer patients, but it is your own responsibility to be sure that you receive the maximum benefits. If you misinterpret your medical insurance coverage and later find that the service is not covered, you are, in many cases, responsible to pay for that service. Therefore, be persistent and ask many questions to find out what is actually covered. Some policies, for example, cover medical equipment, such as hospital beds for in-home care, or prostheses, such as wigs or breast substitutes for mastectomy patients, but they do not display this information prominently in their informational brochures. Sometimes speaking with the employer's benefits coordinator or the customer service department of your insurance plan reveals benefits that are not immediately apparent. Also, be sure your physician verifies the cancer diagnosis to your insurance company so you can obtain maximum benefits.

Prepaid health plans offered by health maintenance organizations (HMOs) usually provide full coverage of physicians' costs. Your physician may also reduce his or her fees to meet your financial needs, but you must inform your physician or the office staff if financial problems arise. Hospital-paid oncologists who work in oncology clinics also will adjust fees through the business office of the hospital. Social service workers attached to these units can intercede with hospital billing offices to get fees reduced and insurance paperwork expedited.

Hospitals built with federal grants must offer a certain amount of free care to their patients. It does not hurt to ask about this potential source of financial help.

If you are in need of special equipment, such as hospital beds for home use or pumps, consider renting these items rather than purchasing them outright. Insurance companies vary in their reimbursement policies, so consult with your insurance representatives or with your local hospital supply companies. The latter will often bill insurance companies directly and advise you about the advantages and disadvantages of renting. Standard durable medical equipment, such as beds, walkers, and commodes, are competitively priced, so it pays to "shop around." Oncology nurses and social workers, as well as health care agencies such as visiting nurses' associations, are good sources of information on fairly priced medical equipment. A quick telephone survey to compare prices will also help you save time and money.

Chemotherapy drugs are very expensive, particularly the newer agents. Insurance companies may cover only part of the cost. You can minimize your out-of-pocket expenses by using clinics and physicians that supply the drugs and bill insurance companies directly. If this is not possible and drugs must be purchased from pharmacies, compare the prices between chain and nonchain pharmacies to save money. Too many patients buy their medications without checking prices in several local pharmacies. Chain pharmacies are not necessarily the cheapest. Pharmacies associated with insurance plans or unions can sometimes supply drugs at the lowest cost. To locate these pharmacies, ask your benefits coordinator at work or check with the member relations department of your insurance plan. Almost all pharmaceutical companies will supply their anticancer drugs at a reduced price or even at no cost to patients who need the drug but are unable to pay for it. Have your oncologist check with the appropriate drug company, if no other affordable source is available.

There are many sources of financial aid, but they usually cover only medical expenses. Living expenses may be the worst problem for families with cancer victims. Not only do the usual expenses such as rent and food continue, but other expenses actually increase, such as the cost of transportation to treatment centers or the need for homemaker services to help a sick mother.

Medicare, HMOs, private commercial insurance, Blue Cross–Blue Shield plans, and Medicaid pay for most cancer care. Benefits available from these plans vary tremendously. It is essential that all available benefits be used, and sometimes it is hard to find someone knowledgeable enough to be aware of all the possibilities. At the "Blues" (Blue Cross, Blue Shield, or their equivalents) and commercial insurance companies, there is usually an administrator or service representative who acts as liaison for the insurance plan, its sponsor (usually an employer), and the patients covered by the plan. This person may be located at the insured's place of employment or at the insurance company itself. If you have questions about your coverage that are not readily answered by plan literature or health care providers, consult these liaison service representatives. If answers are not forthcoming or are incomplete, consult your hospital or HMO social service departments, community health care agencies, or your doctor's billing office. It is very important that benefits you are entitled to are not overlooked during the very stressful period of initial evaluation and treatment for cancer.

Once insurance benefits have been exhausted or noncovered expenses are becoming a financial burden, other sources of aid may be available. For example, local offices of the American Cancer Society or the United Cancer Council may be able to find you help. Various community service agencies and public welfare agencies can sometimes be useful. State public welfare departments, Medicaid, or medical assistance programs run by the state and partially funded by the federal government may help you keep up with medical expenses. Keep in mind that help for a specific problem is usually available, but it may take some telephoning or researching to find it. In the future, national health or catastrophic illness insurance may relieve the financial burden of a cancer illness. (Appendix B contains a list of service agencies that can help you find aid or answer questions.)

If financial aid is not available, ask your doctor about experimental cancer programs, particularly if the treatment plan you both agreed on is proving inadequate (see Chapter 3 for more details about these programs). Often direct or indirect financial support can come from participating in experimental studies. The National Cancer Institute in Bethesda, Maryland, for example, pays for the inpatient care of cancer patients it is studying. Similar programs may exist in your local hospitals and cancer centers. Again, ask your doctor about programs in your area.

Home-Based Cancer Chemotherapy

Before you consider having treatment administered in your home, you must remember, first and foremost, that your family must be willing and *able* to participate in such a program. Usually home-based treatment begins only after initial therapy has been administered in a hospital or an oncology outpatient facility. You, as most patients do, may quickly come to dislike long hospitalizations, traveling to appointments, and having to wait in an outpatient clinic. Your family may want to help you avoid these problems and inconveniences, but they must also be able to provide someone to act as a twenty-four-hour liaison between you and health care providers. Coordination between the various services needed to care for a cancer patient at home is usually provided by social workers or nurses attached to a hospital (including Veterans Administration hospitals), visiting nurse association, private home care agency, or community health facility.

Well before modern hospital facilities were available, patients with cancer were cared for at home. Families worked together to see to every need of these patients. But with the advancements of modern chemotherapy and hospital facilities to deliver specialized cancer care, the advantages of home care were slowly forgotten. Recently, social service agencies and hospitals have combined their efforts and technology to make it possible to treat all but the most seriously ill and unstable cancer patients at home. Home care saves money because you avoid being admitted to the hospital. Many insurance companies pay for home care just as they would for a hospital stay. If you would like to have treatment at home, discuss the possibility with your oncologist. If he or she agrees that home care is appropriate for you, your oncologist will help you make the arrangements.

A major stumbling block to home care developed because of the concern in administering toxic anticancer drugs. The use of these drugs usually required the supervision of an oncologist. A special pump, however, has been designed to deliver the drugs into a permanently implanted catheter, making it possible for specially trained teams of nurses to administer treatment in patients' homes. The drug may be administered either as a "bolus injection," in which a syringe filled with a drug is emptied into the catheter over a period of a few minutes, or as an "infusion," in which the contents of a bag containing the drug are emptied into the catheter over a period of thirty to sixty minutes. (See Chapter 8 for a description of how catheters are implanted.)

Two types of chemotherapy pumps may be used to deliver anticancer drugs into the blood. External pumps are usually worn on a belt and attached to an indwelling catheter that has been inserted into a large vein. A syringe built into the pump unit acts as the reservoir to hold the drug. A battery-powered motor drives the barrel of the syringe. As the barrel moves, it forces liquid out of the syringe, into the catheter, and ultimately into the patient's blood. The second type of pump is more permanent because it is surgically placed under the skin of the chest. To fill the pump, a technician or nurse pierces the skin with a needle and injects the drug into the pump's reservoir. The outflow from the reservoir goes through an indwelling catheter into a large vein. Instead of battery power, the force needed to drive the liquid out of the pump and into the patient's blood is obtained from an elastic membrane stretched during filling of the pump's reservoir. The force of this membrane pressing against the fluid drives it into the catheter and the blood.

Either type of pump is refilled by the intravenous technician during a home visit or at the time of a clinic appointment. Patients using external pumps can obtain a supply of prefilled syringes to deliver a drug over a period of days without the need for outside assistance. Patients may be able to administer the drug themselves, or they may need assistance from family members or trained technicians. A patient's dependence on others for home care help depends entirely on his or her individual circumstances and needs.

If you choose to receive treatment at home, you must have an adequate refrigerator to store your drugs and sterile solutions, a clean area where sterile operations and mixing can be performed, hot water, toilet facilities, and space for family members to sleep while attending you.

You may find that financing home-based chemotherapy is a problem; your insurance may cover only part of the costs. Federal regulations continue to change, but in most cases, cancer patients covered by Medicare who are not expected to live more than six months and need treatment for symptoms or pain control are entitled to 210 days of home care through hospice programs. (Hospices are discussed later in this chapter.) Check through your Social Security Administration offices, hospital social service departments, hospices, home health care agencies, or visiting nurse associations for the latest rules and regulations concerning Medicare reimbursement for home cancer care. Most private insurance plans have added coverage for cancer patients, and this will often pick up the cost of pumps, supplies, and specially trained nurses or technicians you require to administer the prescribed chemotherapy. In any case, it is crucial for you and your family to discuss with your social worker and oncologist your health insurance plan to ensure that full benefits for home care are received.

Home care services are certified by federal agencies, i.e., Medicare, Medicaid, and the Veterans Administration, and by state governments. Other accrediting agencies are: National Home Caring Council, National League for Nursing, American Public Health Association, and the Joint Commission on Accreditation of Health Care Organizations. Home care professionals are tested, certified, and licensed by individual states—a function that varies greatly throughout the United States. A patient can find out if a particular service or home care professional is certified by asking the individual agency, or by checking with the local visiting nurse association or similar cancer service organization. All these certifications have different requirements, and they carry no guarantees. They are valuable only because they recognize the services or professionals as qualified to perform home care. Recommendations from satisfied clients should also help greatly in selecting a home health care provider.

In most cases, it's a good idea to select one agency to coordinate all aspects of your home-based chemotherapy. This agency will provide nurses and equipment, such as hospital beds, commodes, and walkers, and will arrange for delivery of drugs and supplies, blood testing, administration of intravenous drugs, pump maintenance, and catheter care. Homemakers, home health aides, and social workers are often available through these home care programs. Still, remember that your physician will supervise your care, prescribe the chemotherapy drugs, and visit you for routine care, emotional support, or in the event of an emergency. Outpatient oncology units can add extra support to these special efforts, especially if you are able to visit the unit at least once a month.

The following checklist can help you determine whether or not home chemotherapy is feasible for your needs:

____ Do you and your family want to do chemotherapy at home?

____ Does your physician feel that you are a candidate for home care? Is your condition stable, without requiring frequent monitoring and specialized hospital care?

____ Will insurance or other resources cover the cost of home care services?

_____ Is a family member willing and able to act as a twenty-four-hour liaison between you and your care providers?

_____ Is your home set up for care of catheters and intravenous administration of drugs? For example, is there adequate refrigeration, storage space for sterile supplies, and a clean area for sterile operations and mixing of drug solutions?

_____ Are physicians available to visit, supervise chemotherapy, and provide emergency assistance?

_____ Will there be any problems coordinating hospital or clinic care with home care; will your hospital, or another inpatient unit, accept you for admission, if required?

_____ Are the patient's veins suitable for intravenous chemotherapy; can a permanent catheter be implanted?

_____ Is the patient expected to live long enough to justify the time and effort required to set up home chemotherapy?

If these questions are answered satisfactorily, home-based chemotherapy becomes a viable alternative to inpatient or even outpatient clinic care. Many patients remain at home throughout their treatments, visiting the outpatient clinics infrequently for consultations and treatment of complications.

Hospice Programs

The hospice concept is an extension of services previously supplied by home health care agencies such as visiting nurse associations. The hospice program for cancer patients originated in Europe and in the United States in response to more patients' wanting home care during advanced stages of their disease. In the hospice type of treatment, terminally ill patients are usually cared for at home or in homelike institutional facilities. Hospice personnel maintain the patient's comfort and provide emotional support, but they use no "heroic measures" to prolong the patient's life. Many hospices are run by religious organizations, and they all have spiritual and emotional counseling services. Cancer hospice programs deal only with terminally ill cancer patients, and their range of services is generally greater than that previously available through home care agencies. Most patients are expected to remain at home during their terminal illness, but it is possible to switch back to hospital care in the unlikely event it becomes necessary. The hospice coordinates all services, including physician care, nurses, homemakers, and medical equipment rentals. The hospice may also have an inpatient or hospital unit available for patients who cannot, for some reason, have these services delivered at home. Patients generally prefer home-based hospice services over inpatient hospice care. Some hospice programs offer respite programs, during which the patient's care is removed from family members and taken over for a period of time by the hospital or specially trained hospice personnel. This gives responsible family members a chance to rest before resuming care of the patient.

CHAPTER 2

Chemotherapy:
An Overview

Chemotherapy is the use of chemicals to treat cancer. The chemicals may be called drugs, medications, or agents. The chemicals used have a toxic effect on cancerous cells, and the chemotherapy's targets are the cells that make up the tumor. Some drugs are more effective than others against specific types of cancer. The way a particular chemotherapeutic agent works is called its mode of action. Commonly, it prevents cells from multiplying by interfering with the metabolism—processes that maintain life and growth—of the tumor cells.

Treatments are scheduled in cycles, also called courses of therapy. The first drug (or group of drugs) you receive is called first-line therapy. The goal of first-line therapy is usually to cure the cancer. If it is not successful, follow-up treatments may use different drugs as second-line therapy. Second-line therapy is also intended to cure the cancer, but the drug used has not generally been as effective as the first-line drugs in treating your type of cancer, and side effects may be worse.

History of Chemotherapy

The history of modern-day cancer chemotherapy is closely tied to the development of drugs to treat infectious disease. Cancer cells and bacteria are both foreign invaders to the body. Some drugs initially used as antibiotics against bacteria have also been effective against cancer cells. In 1909, Paul Ehrlich produced a drug that cured syphilis. In the 1920s, antibiotics against the *Staphylococcus* type of bacteria—a frequent cause of pus-producing infections and food poisoning—were discovered. In the 1940s, drugs active against malaria were developed in response to the needs of soldiers fighting in World War II. In each of these instances, it was only a matter of time before similar drugs were tried for the treatment of cancer.

One of the earliest forms of chemotherapy, and certainly the most dramatic, evolved from wartime experience with nitrogen mustard. Soldiers exposed to and killed by this gas during combat in World War I suffered severe damage to their bone marrow and lymph nodes. Autopsies later showed that normal cells in these organs had been destroyed. This dramatic observation led scientists in 1947 to try using similar compounds on patients with lymph node cancers (lymphomas). This first attempt at chemotherapy was very successful.

It was not long before related compounds were synthesized and tried, first in animals and then in humans. Some of these drugs, called antimetabolites, interfered with the life processes and duplication of cells. Others were substances extracted from plants with cell-destroying properties. Still others were compounds made from toxic metals, such as platinum. Certain antibiotics, originally tested for their ability to treat infectious diseases, were also found to inhibit the growth of tumors when used on human tumors transplanted into animals. Any drug effective against bacteria is a candidate for trial against cancer cells. Antibiotics successfully used against cancer include actinomycin and daunomycin.

With the introduction of new agents into the treatment of cancer, new strategies were developed to administer them. In the 1960s, the idea of combination chemotherapy or multidrug therapy evolved. Groups of agents, each acting in a slightly different way and with different side effects, were administered to patients in the hope that cancer cells resistant to individual agents would not be able to survive. Today, we know that diseases such as lymphoma, leukemia, and cancers of the testes can be cured with such combinations of drugs.

Once it was clear that combination chemotherapy could successfully treat cancer, it was only a short step to adapting the same method to prevent cancer from recurring. It was already known that cancer cells could escape from the primary site, lie dormant, and then spread to new locations. To prevent this from happening, the tumor was surgically removed and the primary site was exposed to radiation. Combination chemotherapy was then administered in an attempt to destroy any small secondary tumors, leaving the patient free of cancer. Today, this strategy, called adjuvant therapy, is successful, for example, in treating early breast cancer.

It was also in the late 1960s when chemotherapy was first used in conjunction with radiotherapy in what was called "combined modality" treatment. Hodgkin's disease, a type of lymphoma (lymph node cancer), is often treated in this way. Radiotherapy was administered either before or after chemotherapy. The risk of complications, such as the appearance of a second malignancy, was high with this form of therapy. Nevertheless, it did appear to increase the number of patients considered to be long-term survivors or cures. The use of combined modality treatment led to development of today's cancer treatment teams. Surgeons, radiotherapists, and oncologists (cancer specialists) now work together to plan and carry out treatment strategies designed for individual patients.

Drugs Commonly Used for Chemotherapy

Your oncologist can administer chemotherapy using one drug (single-drug therapy) or a group of drugs chosen to work together (multidrug therapy). Many tumors quickly become resistant or unresponsive to one drug, but they cannot resist the different effects of multiple drugs acting together. As the disease progresses to advanced stages and you receive more chemotherapy, you may find that the tumors may resist even multiple drugs.

The way the drug is administered is called the route:

- IV = intravenous
- IM = intramuscular
- PO = per OS (by mouth)
- SC = subcutaneous (under the skin)
- Topical = applied to the skin
- Intracavitary = injected into the chest or abdominal cavity.

Cost ranges are as follows:

- High = $500 to $1,000 per cycle
- Moderate = $100 to $500 per cycle
- Low = $20 to $100 per cycle
- If a drug has not been FDA approved, it may be available free as part of a clinical study. These drugs are listed as "Investigational." Recently, however, the FDA has allowed manufacturers to charge for non-FDA-approved drugs that are about to be approved and are being used compassionately.

Drug Combinations Commonly Used for Chemotherapy

Chemotherapy may utilize combination agents containing several drugs. It is impossible to include all combinations, but page 45 lists those most commonly used to treat lymphoma and Hodgkin's disease.

How Chemotherapy Works with Other Cancer Treatments

Other prescription drugs may play an important role in your treatment in addition to the necessary chemotherapeutic agents listed above. These include antibiotics to treat infections and sedatives to help you sleep. You may also receive transfusions of whole blood or blood products (plasma or platelets) as supportive treatment to replace red cells if you are anemic or platelets if you develop bleeding problems. Rarely, anticoagulants (e.g., heparin) are given to prevent blood clots, or thrombolytic enzymes (e.g., streptokinase or t-PA) may be used to dissolve clots that have already formed.

Sometimes a patient needs to receive a bone marrow transplant from a healthy donor or from cells taken from the patient's own marrow prior to chemotherapy (see Chapter 8). Such transplants are common in certain cancer treatments.

Certain terms are used to indicate how a particular chemotherapy relates to other cancer treatments:

• If chemotherapy is expected to improve the effectiveness of the other treatment types in destroying the cancer, it is called adjuvant or adjunctive therapy. Adjuvant therapy, therefore, adds to the effectiveness of surgery and radiation for certain types of cancer (see Chapter 5).

• If surgery, radiation, or earlier chemotherapy fails, further chemotherapy may be given in a last-ditch effort to destroy tumor cells and improve quality of life. This is called salvage therapy.

• Sometimes all possible treatment types are unsuccessful and chemotherapy is given to relieve symptoms or slow down the progress of the disease, without any hope of a cure. This is called palliative therapy. Such treatments can help many patients with hard-to-treat cancers by improving their quality of life (see Chapter 6).

Administering Chemotherapy

Many medical procedures are followed during chemotherapy. Some of these procedures are used to diagnose the cancer, evaluate the extent or stage of disease, and monitor the effectiveness of treatment. Other procedures are used for the actual administration of the chemotherapy.

Chemotherapy Agents*

Name	Brand Name	Side Effects	Route	Cost	Cancers Treated
5-Azacytidine	none	Bleeding, infection, diarrhea, mouth sores, nerve pain, water retention, vein inflammation (phlebitis) at injection site	IV	Investigational	Acute leukemia
Aspariginase	Elspar	Drowsiness, fever, chills, joint pain, vomiting, stomach pain, bleeding, mouth sores, problem pregnancy, inflammation of pancreas	IM, IV	Moderate	Acute leukemia
Bleomycin	Blenoxane	Fever, chills, shortness of breath, cough, mouth sores, darkening or thickening of skin, rash, vomiting, diarrhea, weight loss, pain at site of injection, vein inflammation (phlebitis)	IM, IV	Moderate	Lymphoma, head and neck, testes, lung
Busulfan	Myleran	Fever, chills, sore throat, bleeding, shortness of breath, skin darkening, fatigue, weakness, weight loss, false-positive Pap smears, infertility, second malignancy, problem pregnancy	PO	Low	Chronic leukemia
Carboplatin	Paraplatin	Low blood counts, vomiting, nervous system problems, kidney problems, loss of hearing, allergic reactions	IV	High	Lymphoma, ovarian, bladder, lung, testes, head and neck
Carmustine, BCNU	BiCNU	Sores at infusion site, cough, fever, chills, sore throat, shortness of breath, bleeding, mouth sores, vomiting	IV	Moderate	Lymphoma, brain tumors, myeloma

*This alphabetical list is adapted and modified from *Chemotherapy and You: A Guide to Self-help During Treatment,* published by the U.S. Department of Health and Human Services as NIH Publication NO. 85-1136 and is available by telephoning 1-800-4-CANCER or writing the Office of Cancer Communications, National Cancer Institute, Building 31, Room 10A18, Bethesda, MD 20205.

Name	Brand Name	Side Effects	Route	Cost	Cancers Treated
Chlorambucil	Leukeran	Fever, chills, sore throat, mouth sores, bleeding, skin rash, yellowing of eyes and skin, infertility, problem pregnancy, second malignancy	PO	Low	Lymphoma, chronic leukemia
Cisplatin, Cisplatinum	Platinol	Immediate wheezing and face swelling, sores at site of injection, loss of hearing, vomiting, low urine output (kidney failure), nerve inflammation (neuritis), problem pregnancy	IV	High	Lymphoma, ovarian, bladder, lung, testes, head and neck
Cyclophosphamide	Cytoxan, Neosar	Bladder irritation, blood in urine, fever, chills, bleeding, loss of hair, vomiting, loss of menstrual periods (infertility), second malignancy, problem pregnancy	IV, PO	Low	Lymphoma, leukemia, ovarian, lung, testes, breast, multiple myeloma, mycosis fungoides, tumors of retina, sarcoma
Cytarabine, Cytosine arabinoside, Ara-C	Cytosar-U	Fever, chills, sore throat, bleeding, rash, mouth sores, dizziness, difficulty walking, liver inflammation (jaundice), kidney failure, vomiting, problem pregnancy	IV, IM	Moderate	Acute leukemia
Dacarbazine, DTIC	DTIC-Dome	Sores at site of injection, fever, flushing, chills, sore throat, vomiting, bleeding, mouth sores	IV	Moderate	Melanoma, lymphoma, sarcoma

37

Name	Brand Name	Side Effects	Route	Cost	Cancers Treated
Dactinomycin, Actinomycin D	Cosmegen	Immediate wheezing, severe sores at site of injection, fever, chills, sore throat, bleeding, mouth sores, vomiting, skin darkening, hair loss, liver failure (jaundice), second malignancy, problem pregnancy	IV	Low	Tumors of the placenta, sarcoma, Wilm's tumor, testes
Daunorubicin, Daunomycin	Cerubidine	Red urine, heart problems (including irregular beats and heart failure), fluid retention, shortness of breath, sores at site of infusion, fever, chills, sore throat, bleeding, mouth sores, vomiting, hair loss, rash, liver problems (at higher doses), problem pregnancy	IV	Moderate	Acute leukemia
Deoxyco-fomycin	Pentostatin	Vomiting, rash, liver and kidney problems	IV	Investigational	Hairy cell leukemia
Doxorubicin	Adriamycin	Red urine, heart problems (including irregular rhythm and heart failure), fluid retention, shortness of breath, sores at site of injection, fever, chills, sore throat, bleeding, mouth sores, vomiting, diarrhea, hair loss, skin reaction (after radiotherapy), problem pregnancy	IV	Moderate	Breast, lymphoma, leukemia, ovarian, lung, bladder, head and neck, pancreas, sarcoma, testes, stomach
Estramustine	Emcyt	Headaches, loss of coordination, calf pain, shortness of breath, vision changes, breast tenderness, nausea, rash, fever, second malignancy, problem pregnancy	PO	High	Prostate

Name	Brand Name	Side Effects	Route	Cost	Cancers Treated
Etoposide, VP-16	Vepesid	Bleeding, infection, nausea, aftertaste, vomiting, hair loss, nervous symptoms, skin reaction (after radiotherapy), second malignancy, problem pregnancy, severe allergic reaction (rarely)	IV, PO	Moderate	Lymphoma, Kaposi's sarcoma, lung, leukemia, testes, brain, tumor of placenta
Floxuridine	FUDR	Vomiting, diarrhea, fever, chills, mouth sores, bleeding, liver inflammation, nervous symptoms (loss of balance)	IV	Moderate	Colon
Fluorouracil, 5FU	Adrucil, Efudex	Vomiting, diarrhea, fever, chills, mouth sores, bleeding, skin darkening, hair loss, sores at site of injection, very low white blood cell counts	IV, PO	Low	Colon, pancreas, breast, head and neck, ovarian, skin, stomach, bladder
Hexamethyl-melamine	none	Vomiting, nervous symptoms, seizures	PO, topical	Investigational	Ovarian
Hydroxyurea	Hydrea	Vomiting, diarrhea, fever, chills, mouth sores, bleeding, headache, confusion, skin reaction (after radiotherapy), problem pregnancy	PO	Moderate	Chronic leukemia
Ifosfamide	Ifex	Similar to cyclophosphamide. Bladder irritation, blood in urine, fever, chills, bleeding, hair loss, vomiting, loss of menstrual periods (infertility), second malignancy, problem pregnancy	IV	Moderate	Sarcomas, breast, lung, lymphoma, ovarian, testes

39

Name	Brand Name	Side Effects	Route	Cost	Cancers Treated
Interferon	Intron A, Roferon A	Fever, chills, joint pain, low blood counts, fatigue, weight loss	IV, SC	High	Hairy cell leukemia, chronic myelocytic leukemia, Kaposi's sarcoma, lymphoma, myeloma, melanoma, kidney, breast, bladder
Leucovorin	Wellcovorin, Leucovorin-Calcium	Allergic reactions	IV, IM, PO	Moderate	Colon, antidote for methotrexate toxicity
Leuprolide	Lupron	Hot flashes, breast tenderness, nervous symptoms, heart problems, vomiting, constipation, blood in urine, impotency, lung or kidney problems, rash, hair loss, itch, fever, fluid retention	SC	High	Prostate
Lomustine, CCNU	CeeNU	Vomiting, diarrhea, fever, chills, mouth sores, bleeding, confusion, skin darkening, shortness of breath, second malignancy	PO	Moderate	Brain, lymphoma
m-AMSA	Amsacrine	Nausea, vomiting, bleeding, infection, vein inflammation (phlebitis), heart problems	IV	Investigational	Acute leukemia

Name	Brand Name	Side Effects	Route	Cost	Cancers Treated
Mechlore-thamine, Nitrogen mustard	Mustargen	Immediate wheezing, sores at site of injection, vomiting, diarrhea, fever, chills, mouth sores, bleeding, infertility, liver inflammation (jaundice), hearing loss, second malignancy, problem pregnancy	IV	Low	Lymphoma
Megesterol	Megace	Vein inflammation (phlebitis), hair loss, fluid retention, problem pregnancy	PO	Moderate	Prostate, breast
Melphalan, Phenylalanine mustard, L-PAM	Alkeran	Skin rash, vomiting, diarrhea, fever, chills, mouth sores, bleeding, second malignancy, problem pregnancy	PO	Moderate	Myeloma, chronic leukemia
Mercapto-purine, 6MP	Purinethol	Vomiting, diarrhea, fever, chills, mouth sores, bleeding, liver inflammation (jaundice), second malignancy, problem pregnancy. Lower dose should be used if patient is receiving allopurinol. Avoid alcohol (makes side effects worse).	PO	Moderate	Acute leukemia
Methotrexate	Mexate, Folex	Liver problems (avoid alcohol), kidney problems, vomiting, diarrhea, fever, chills, mouth sores, bleeding, seizures, headache, confusion, sensitivity to sunlight (sunburn easily), hair loss, infertility, problem pregnancy	IV, IM, PO	Moderate	Leukemia, breast, head and neck, lymphoma, sarcoma, mycosis fungoides

41

Name	Brand Name	Side Effects	Route	Cost	Cancers Treated
Mitomycin	Mutamycin	Vomiting, diarrhea, fever, chills, mouth sores, bleeding, blood in urine, sores at site of injection, kidney problems (fluid retention), second malignancy, problem pregnancy	IV	High	Breast, stomach
Mitotane, o,p-DDD	Lysodren	Drowsiness, worsens sedative effects of alcohol and other drugs, vomiting, diarrhea, blood in urine, wheezing, shortness of breath	PO	Moderate	Adrenal
Mitoxantrone	Novantrone	Similar to adriamycin and daunomycin, but less risk of heart problems. Fever, chills, sore throat, bleeding, mouth sores, vomiting, diarrhea	IV	Moderate	Breast, leukemia, lymphoma
Plicamycin	Mithracin, Mithramycin	Bleeding, vomiting, confusion, depression, fever, chills, mouth sores	IV, IM	Moderate	Testes
Prednisone	Deltasone, Meticorten, Orasone, Serapred	Diabetes, acne, bleeding from stomach ulcers, high blood pressure, leg swelling, depression, nervousness, confusion, poor healing, weight gain, severe infections, low blood pressure when treatment stops, muscle weakness	IV, IM, PO	Low	Lymphoma, leukemia

Name	Brand Name	Side Effects	Route	Cost	Cancers Treated
Procarbazine	Matulane, Natulan	High blood pressure, reactions to alcohol and aged foods (such as cheese), reactions to over-the-counter medications, drowsiness, vomiting, diarrhea, fever, chills, mouth sores, bleeding, liver inflammation (jaundice), confusion, headache, fainting, skin darkening, irregular menstrual periods, problem pregnancy	PO	Low	Lymphoma, brain
Streptozocin	Zanosar	Sores at site of injection, nervousness, shakiness, chills, cold sweats, drowsiness, hunger (low blood sugar), fast pulse, fever, chills, liver inflammation (jaundice), sore throat, fluid retention, kidney failure, second malignancy, problem pregnancy	IV	Moderate	Pancreas, islet cell
Tamoxifen	Nolvadex	Hot flashes, vaginal bleeding, bone pain, fluid retention, high calcium levels in the blood, problem pregnancy	PO	Moderate	Breast, prostate
Teniposide, VM-26	none	Severe allergic reaction (rare), bleeding, infection, nausea, vomiting, hair loss, nervous system problems, second malignancy, problem pregnancy	IV	Investigational	Brain, lymphoma, lung, leukemia, testes
Thioguanine, 6TG	Thioguanine	Bleeding, infection, anemia, liver problems (including jaundice), higher uric acid levels in the blood, second malignancy, problem pregnancy	PO	Moderate	Acute leukemia
ThioTEPA	ThioTEPA	Anemia, bleeding, infection, second malignancy, birth defects	IV, Intracavitary	Moderate	Breast, bladder, malignant effusions, ovary

43

Name	Brand Name	Side Effects	Route	Cost	Cancers Treated
Vinblastine	Velban, Velbe	Sores at site of injection, fever, chills, mouth sores, bleeding, jaw pain, nervous system problems (double or blurred vision, droopy eyelids, tingling in toes and fingers, dizziness), hair loss, infertility, problem pregnancy	IV	Moderate	Breast, Kaposi's sarcoma, tumors of placenta, testes, lymphoma, mycosis fungoides
Vincristine	Oncovin	Constipation, stomach cramps, sores at site of infection, nervous system problems (double or blurred vision, droopy eyelids, tingling in toes and fingers, dizziness, hallucinations), difficult urination, fluid retention, fever, chills, sore throat, jaw pain, mouth sores, bleeding, hair loss, infertility, second malignancy, problem pregnancy	IV	Moderate	Brain, breast, lymphoma, leukemia, lung, sarcoma, Wilm's tumor
Vindesine	Eldisine	Sores at site of injection, bleeding, nervous system problems	IV	Investigational	Breast, lung, leukemia, lymphoma

44

Combination Chemotherapy for Lymphoma

Combination Name	Cyclophosphamide	Vincristine	Prednisone	Dexamethasone	Adriamycin	Procarbazine	Bleomycin	Methotrexate with Rescue	Cytosine arabinoside	Etoposide (VP-16)	Nitrogen mustard
COP	•	•	•								
CHOP	•	•	•		•						
C-MOPP	•	•	•			•					
BACOP	•	•	•		•		•				
COMLA	•	•						•	•		
PRO MACE-MOPP	•	•	•		•	•		•		•	•
M-BACOD	•	•		•	•		•	•			
COP-BLAM	•	•	•		•	•	•				
MACOP-B	•	•	•		•		•	•			

Combination Chemotherapy for Hodgkin's Disease

	Nitrogen Mustard	Vincristine	Procarbazine	Prednisone	Adriamycin	Bleomycin	Vinblastine	DTIC
MOPP	•	•	•	•				
ABVD					•	•	•	•
MOPP/ABVD	•	•	•	•	•	•	•	•

Diagnosis, Evaluation, and Monitoring

A number of tests and procedures are done periodically to diagnose cancer, to evaluate the success or failure of treatment, and to monitor the patient's condition. The tests are the same; the purpose of the tests will vary according to the times when they are done.

Before starting chemotherapy, patients usually undergo a number of tests to confirm the diagnosis of cancer and to evaluate their condition. A physical examination is done by the physician or oncologist to obtain a medical history of the patient; check the heart, lungs, and blood pressure; feel the tumor; or otherwise look for signs and symptoms of the disease.

Cancers in the lung, bones, or elsewhere are diagnosed with X rays or other imaging procedures that use radioactive substances called isotopes. Computerized techniques called CAT scans are used for viewing with great detail soft tissue that would be invisible to ordinary X rays. Mammograms are specialized X rays for detecting tumors in the breast. Magnetic resonance imaging, MRI, is a relatively new technique for diagnosing cancer and for showing how far it has spread. MRI uses the fact that atoms in magnetic fields have different physical characteristics—resonances—to produce images of internal body structures, such as the bones, brain, or lymph nodes. MRI does not use X rays and, in some cases, is preferred over X rays because it gives clearer images.

Many tests are performed by technologists in a laboratory managed by a pathologist, a physician specializing in diagnosis and analysis of specimens. These tests are most often done on blood samples. Your blood is made up of three types of cells (red blood cells, white blood cells, and platelets) suspended in a liquid called plasma (after clotting, plasma is called serum). A cell count indicates the presence of anemia, infection, or potential bleeding problems, all of which are potential side effects of certain chemotherapeutic drugs. Patients are often concerned about their white blood cell counts, since chemotherapy frequently causes a decrease in the number of white cells, thereby increasing the risk of serious infection.

A culture test of the patient's blood, sputum, or other body fluids indicates whether disease-causing organisms, such as bacteria or viruses, are present. Your doctor may also test the levels of certain other substances (markers) in the plasma or serum for indications of particular types of cancer. Other tests measure substances that show how well certain organs, like the liver or kidney, are functioning.

A biopsy is a procedure in which a sample of living tissue from an organ or suspected tumor is taken for laboratory analysis. A bone marrow aspiration, for example, is a type of biopsy in which a specimen of bone marrow is taken from inside a bone, often the pelvic bone at the hip. The technologist or pathologist prepares the biopsy specimen and then observes the cells through a microscope to determine whether they are malignant (cancerous) or benign (noncancerous).

Administration Procedures

The way chemotherapy is administered involves a variety of factors, including: the treatment plan, what drug(s) will be used, how much should be given and when, and how the drug(s) should be given.

Treatment plan. Doctors, nurses, and technologists all play a role in your overall care during chemotherapy, as with any other medical treatment. The physician who decides the treatment plan (also called the program, regimen, or protocol) may be from any of a number of specialties, depending on the type of cancer you have, the institution providing the treatments, or your own preferences. Physicians specializing in internal medicine treat diseases of the internal organs by noninvasive, that is nonsurgical, techniques that include medication, diet, and other life-style changes. By contrast, surgeons treat disease by invasive techniques that repair, replace, or remove organs or tissue.

Ultimately, however, the decision to administer chemotherapy lies with the patient. Before any program begins, the physician will discuss the treatment fully with you and your family, explaining risks, potential benefits, and alternatives, and then obtain written permission (informed consent) to proceed with the treatment (see Appendix A).

What drug(s) will be used. Chemotherapy is an extremely complex area of medicine. New chemotherapeutic agents and new methods of using existing agents are being developed constantly. A single drug or combination of drugs will be selected by the oncologist, based on his or her experience and knowledge of the drug, the disease, and the patient's specific needs.

How much should be given and when. The amount of a specific drug or combination of drugs that will be given is called the dose or dosage. Dosages may be in milligrams, milliliters, or some other unit of measure. The timing of doses is called the dosing schedule. Schedules use such terms as continuous (uninterrupted); intermittent (with breaks); one, two, or three times daily; or as needed.

Chemotherapy is given in cycles—outlined in the signed treatment plan—in which patients receive a certain drug or a combination of drugs over a period of time. They are then given a waiting period before receiving another cycle of the same or different drug or combination of drugs. The waiting period allows time for the drug to work and gives the patient a chance to recuperate before the next cycle begins. An average cycle takes two to four weeks.

How the drug(s) should be given. There are five common ways chemotherapeutic drugs can be administered. The method used depends on many factors, including the nature of the drug, the location of the cancer, and the condition of the patient.

1. The drug may be taken orally (by mouth). This is the most convenient way to administer a drug. When a drug is taken orally, it passes through the stomach, digestive system, and ultimately throughout the entire body. In the process, it is altered by digestive enzymes and other chemicals. These alterations can ultimately make the drug less effective or more easily excreted from the body.

2. Generally, chemotherapy is given by injection into the body through a needle and syringe. An injection into muscle tissue is called an intramuscular injection. This method allows the drug to be absorbed slowly into the blood, with little or no alteration, but it can be irritating and painful.

3. More commonly, the drug is injected into a vein. Intravenous (IV) injections allow the drug to enter the patient's blood quickly and unchanged by digestive processes.

4. If the drug needs to be administered frequently over a long period of time, it is common to leave the needle in place and install a catheter (plastic tube) between the needle and the reservoir, which may be a bottle, bag, or a pump for controlling drug flow. A stopcock on the catheter is used to shut off the flow between treatment intervals. This method of administering the agent slowly into the vein is called an intravenous (IV) infusion. A temporary catheter is removed after the treatment is over, whereas a permanent one is kept in place between treatments. An indwelling catheter is surgically implanted under the patient's skin for use in subsequent treatments. A catheter can also be fitted with an outflow device, enabling blood sampling between treatments.

5. A final method of administering chemotherapy is called instillation. This technique delivers the agent directly into the affected area. This is often painful, so most patients receive local anesthesia before treatment. It is usually performed with a needle inserted through the skin into the affected body cavity. Tumors treated in this way include advanced ovarian cancers and advanced lung cancers, which are often difficult to treat with drugs that pass through the bloodstream. The advantage of this method is that the side effects are generally reduced, because the agent works directly on the tumor without passing through the rest of the body.

Evaluating the Success of Chemotherapy

Chemotherapy has some major limitations. Because it is generally toxic to normal cells, especially rapidly dividing ones, as well as to malignant cells, it causes serious side effects. Such side effects include nausea, vomiting, hair loss, and infertility. Mouth sores may be caused by its effects on mucous membranes on the inside of the mouth and gums.

Another common side effect is bone marrow suppression—that is, the bone marrow cells no longer develop normally. This may result in a number of problems: the patient may become anemic because there are not enough red cells to carry oxygen; there may not be enough white blood cells to fight off infection; or the lack of platelets can prevent clotting and cause unnecessary blood loss.

Despite these limitations, chemotherapy can be effective if the goals of therapy are well defined and followed. You and your physician should remain focused on the original expectations of the benefits you will gain from using a selected drug program, whether it is to cure the cancer, to reduce the size of the tumor, to stop or slow down the spread of cancer, to increase the effectiveness of surgery or radiation, or to relieve symptoms.

Chemotherapy is considered successful if it meets or exceeds these expectations. The term *cure* has a different meaning with cancer than with other diseases. Some patients do remain totally free of cancer after treatment. However, a cure more often means long-term survival. For example, a patient may be considered cured if he or she remains free of disease for five years.

If the tumor is removed or reduced by surgery, chemotherapy, and/or radiation, the patient may appear to be cured. This is called remission. Some tumors are said to be persistent if they resist treatment. If a tumor responds to treatment and then comes back, it is called recurrent. The recurrence of cancer in a patient who was considered cured or in remission is called a relapse. If the patient's condition worsens, it is called exacerbation of the disease. As the disease progresses, organs can fail and other diseases can result, causing the patient's condition to deteriorate even further. These subsequent disease processes are called complications.

Chemotherapy is continuously evolving, however, and new agents are constantly being developed to help lessen the odds of recurrence or exacerbation.

CHAPTER 3

Development and Testing

Development of Cancer Drugs

Before new drugs become available for general use they must undergo a long period of development and clinical trial—a process that is costly and often takes three to five years or more. Items contributing to the high cost of development and trials include: hospital facilities and services; equipment; drug manufacturing; patient support expenses; liability insurance; and specialized personnel to monitor trials, analyze data, write and submit reports, and provide consultation. Today's trials are almost exclusively funded by pharmaceutical companies and carried out at cancer centers. The trials are highly regulated, and information to the public is tightly controlled. The reason for this is to protect the confidentiality of participating patients and centers, to block intrusions into the way the trial is conducted, and to prevent the publication of premature information.

Anticancer drugs, likewise, must undergo lengthy tests and evaluations to satisfy strict FDA requirements. This process is more difficult when testing anticancer drugs than, say, antibiotics. A new antibiotic's value becomes apparent because it actually can halt severe bacterial infections and seldom causes serious side effects. In contrast, a "successful" chemotherapeutic agent may not cure a disease; at best it may prolong survival.

Despite these limitations, anticancer agents are expensive. To understand why, let's trace how these drugs make their way into general use, why so few drugs are available for cancer chemotherapy, and how patients may become involved in experimental studies.

Discovery and Animal Testing

New drugs for cancer clinical trials come from at least five different sources: the synthetic chemical industry, antibiotic research, modification of existing anticancer drugs by the pharmaceutical industry, biochemical research, and accidental discovery.

Forty years ago, the major source of anticancer drugs was the synthetic chemical industry. New chemicals developed for commercial use were tested for any cancer-destroying properties that might make them valuable as chemotherapeutic agents.

Antibiotic research has become another important source of anticancer drugs. Adriamycin, for example, was originally developed as an antibiotic obtained from soil bacteria. During development, it was screened not only for activity against bacteria and viruses but also for anticancer effects. Adriamycin binds to nucleic acid in the cell nucleus, preventing the cell from reproducing. It is no longer used as an antibiotic. Scientists can vary the conditions under which soil bacteria grow to develop new and different antibiotics, all of which are ultimately tested for anticancer activity.

Another productive source is modification of existing anticancer drugs. By altering the chemical structure of a "parent" drug, scientists can develop a whole family of anticancer drugs, each member developed to fight certain types of cancer while reducing side effects. A good example is the family of drugs made from organic compounds of platinum, a type of metal that is toxic to cancer cells.

Biochemical research also provides a limited number of anticancer agents. For example, interferon, a chemical occurring naturally in normal cells, was originally discovered and purified in biochemical laboratories that were studying how cells defend themselves against viruses. When large quantities of interferon became available, scientists discovered its anticancer activity. It is now being used to treat certain cancers of the blood and lymph nodes.

Interestingly, most anticancer agents have resulted from accidental discovery. By chance, a scientist notices that a certain chemical destroys cells. Further testing is performed to confirm if the chemical might be useful as an anticancer agent. Nitrogen mustard, one of the original anticancer drugs, is a good example of an accidental discovery.

Ten thousand chemicals are tested each year for their potential anticancer properties. Animal testing is the first step in determining whether the drug might be effective against cancer. Ideally, drugs would be tested immediately on human tumors transplanted into animals. Because of the time and expense involved, however, it is not possible to try all these agents in living animals. Therefore, so-called antineoplastic (anticancer) drug screens are used to evaluate whether a chemical warrants testing in animals. The common screens use cells removed from human cancers and cultured (allowed to live and grow) in nutrient-containing liquid broth. White blood cells from patients or animals with leukemia (cancer of the blood) are commonly used to make these cultures. The test drug is added to a small quantity of the cultured broth. If the broth contains fewer cells after the test drug is added, then it is likely that the drug has anticancer properties.

Promising drugs are then rescreened on mice with tumors. The tumors may be naturally present in the animals or they may be induced by using cancer-causing chemicals or by injecting cancerous cells taken from tumors in human patients into the animal. Regardless of how the tumor is caused, researchers inject the test drug into the diseased animals and look for any destructive effect on the tumor.

The use of cultures and animals to screen potential agents only begins the process. If screening tests show that the drug is potentially useful as an anticancer agent, a whole series of tests must be performed to learn about the drug's side effects. These tests, again carried out in mice and other animals, are aimed to show what organ(s) are affected by the drug. First, tissue samples are taken from every organ in the body of a test animal. The samples are carefully examined for harmful effects the drugs may have on the structure of the organ. Every system in the animal's body—such as circulatory and respiratory—is then tested for side effects. At this stage of testing, scientists also determine how well and how fast the drug is absorbed into the blood if it is taken by mouth, and how much of the drug reaches various organs. The emphasis at this stage of testing is safety. It is important to use animals first to predict where problems are likely to arise when the drug is eventually tried on humans.

Often "higher" animals such as monkeys are ultimately used for testing. Monkeys and related animals are classified as primates. They are the most highly developed order of animals, and since they are closely related to humans, their reactions may better predict how effective and safe the drug will be in humans. Despite these precautions, however, it is not unusual for unexpected, and sometimes severe, side effects to occur once human testing begins.

Human Trials

Phase I. At this stage, drugs that have had success during animal testing are tried on human cancer patients. So-called Phase I trials are designed and focused to explore only the safety, side effects, and dosing problems for the new, untried agent. Although records are kept of any antitumor responses to the drug, the primary emphasis is on the safety of the patient. The drug is tried in different doses, at different time intervals, and by different routes of administration, such as oral or intravenous. Careful records are kept of any side effects. The goal is to determine the maximum dose that can be given with acceptable side effects.

Acceptable side effects are controllable and reparable. They include: some degree of bone marrow suppression, causing a temporary decrease in red cells, white cells, and platelets; controllable nausea, vomiting, and diarrhea; and hair loss. Unacceptable side effects are irreparable or even life threatening. These include: severe bone marrow suppression, causing life-threatening decreases in blood cells and platelets; severe liver or kidney damage; and uncontrollable vomiting or diarrhea. Any side effect, however, may be considered acceptable if it occurs only rarely during human trials.

Phase II. Trials at this stage are designed to find out specifically which types of cancers respond to the drug. With the information obtained from Phase I trials, scientists will treat a large number of patients with different tumors in the hope of defining which ones are susceptible to the drug. Patients with cancers of the lung, pancreas, and kidney are the most common participants in Phase II trials, since theirs are common cancers that cannot be successfully treated with currently available drugs.

Your oncologist is generally aware of drugs that are in Phase I and Phase II testing. He or she will advise you if you might benefit by entering one of these trials.

Phase III. Finally, in Phase III, drugs shown to be effective against certain tumor types are compared with older agents with known effectiveness to determine if the newer drug is more beneficial or, at least, less toxic. These comparisons often require actual clinical trials, but researchers can also determine the drug's effectiveness by making a "historical" comparison. That is, they examine patients' histories to compare the effect of the new drug with the results other patients have realized when treated with drugs already developed and in use.

If the new drug is to be approved by the Food and Drug Administration (FDA), all human trials, in turn, must be cleared with the FDA and performed under the sponsorship of a hospital or cancer center. To receive FDA clearance, each investigator (i.e., each physician overseeing a trial) submits all information about how the drug is manufactured, potential side effects, animal testing data, and results of any human studies that other investigators may have performed inside or outside the United States.

This same information is also submitted to the sponsoring institution for consideration by a committee concerned with drug trials that require human subjects (patients participating in trials are called "subjects"). This committee is made up not only of physicians but also laypersons with an interest in protecting the rights of patients undergoing treatment with potentially dangerous drugs. The hospital or cancer center committee concerned with human experimentation must prove that the following safeguards are in place before human trials can begin:

• The voluntary consent of the subject is essential. Patients must be adequately informed, orally and usually in writing, about risks and benefits. They should also be aware that they may withdraw from the trial at any time, without interference with the rest of their care.

• Human subjects can be used only if there is no other way to obtain the information.

• All basic scientific data, from animal and human studies, must be made available to the committee.

• Unnecessary risks should not be taken, especially if death or severe disability might result. These risks might include: high doses of drugs without prior testing in animals and humans, use of drugs that have shown a high incidence of unacceptable side effects, or poor supervision of the trial itself by the physician in charge or by the sponsoring organization.

• If there is reason to believe that the trial will fail or that risks are likely without any benefit, then the trial must be discontinued. Risk and benefit must be balanced, so that less risk is taken where the potential benefit is small.

• Adequate facilities and qualified physicians must be available to care for and protect the subjects.

A number of institutions sponsor new anticancer drug development. These centers include the National Cancer Institute in Bethesda, Maryland; Memorial Sloan-Kettering Cancer Center in New York City; University of Texas M. D. Anderson Cancer Center in Houston; Roswell Park Memorial Institute in Buffalo; and others. Groups of hospitals in various parts of the United States often combine their resources and patients to do cooperative trials. These trials involve large numbers of patients treated similarly by different hospitals and physicians. With careful supervision, cooperative trials often yield useful data. They usually involve drugs that show exceptional promise on first screening.

FDA Approval for General Use

After all human studies have been completed, the FDA makes a final decision about approving the agent for general use. Often, approval is given only for certain types of cancers and at specified doses and frequency. Pharmaceutical companies are prohibited from promoting unapproved uses of the drug. In practice, however, once a drug is approved it can be used to treat, in a reasonable fashion, any cancer and in combination with any other approved drugs.

Even after the drug receives approval, both the FDA and the sponsoring pharmaceutical company continue to monitor side effects of the newly released drug. Despite careful initial evaluation, unexpected side effects generally occur when the drug is used in large numbers of patients.

Some drugs have never received official FDA approval, yet they have proven effective against specific types of tumors and have a known and manageable degree of toxicity. There are many reasons why their approval is pending. Sometimes administrative paperwork delays the final approval, but most often, the drugs' effectiveness and safety have not been demonstrated to the satisfaction of the FDA. In this case, further trials or analysis of data is necessary before approval. At times, a drug may be approved for treating one type of tumor; although effective against another type, it still awaits approval for its second "indication." In all these cases, a physician can use the drugs anyway, but sometimes insurance companies will not pay for experimental or non-FDA-approved use of drugs.

Drugs awaiting approval by the FDA are available through the manufacturer or the National Cancer Institute's Division of Cancer Treatment. Oncologists can obtain the drugs for use in clinical studies, for "compassionate" use in patients who do not respond to conventional drug therapy, or for patients with cancers for which there is no effective FDA-approved agent.

Research, Clinical Trials, and the Patient

The three phases of drug testing in humans, then, are as follows: Phase I trials study primarily what doses should be used, how often the drug should be given, and what side effects may be expected. Phase II finds out which diseases are likely to respond. Phase III compares the new treatment with older agents and therapies. Discuss with your doctor whether or not you should participate in clinical trials during any of these three phases.

Choosing to Enter a Trial

Generally speaking, it is best to start treatment with standard therapy (because it is most likely to work) before considering a clinical trial of a new drug. Consider participating in a clinical trial only when standard therapy is not available or is not particularly effective.

In the chapters on specific cancer applications (Chapters 5 and 6), I point out situations wherein experimental treatment seems worth the risks. Nevertheless, there may be strong reasons *not* to participate in a clinical trial. These include:

• There may be a large risk of uncomfortable side effects. Your doctor may be able to anticipate side effects by using the data from other related drugs known to cause side effects or earlier studies that indicate what side effects are likely to occur.
• There may be little expected benefit. Animal studies may show only minor reduction in tumor size, or results may be ambiguous.
• If a new drug is available on a compassionate-use basis, there may be no need to take part in a trial to receive the drug.
• In order for a study to be valid, some participants receive standard therapy, rather than the experimental drug. The patient

may not want to risk being randomized into a group that does not include the experimental drug.

• Travel expenses and living expenses may be too high. Although the treatment is often free, living and travel expenses are not usually covered by the study or by insurance.

Despite these concerns, there are positive reasons to participate in experimental studies:

• There may be no other effective treatment.
• Experts in the treatment of certain cancers often will not treat with new drugs outside a clinical trial. They, and the FDA, feel that only by scientifically studying new drugs under controlled conditions can advances toward cancer cures be made. Patients seeking the advice of these experts will be expected to enroll in clinical studies.
• Some patients feel they have nothing to lose by trying a new drug as part of a clinical trial. The studies will also help other cancer patients by giving investigators the opportunity to evaluate the benefits and side effects of these new agents.

How Trials Work

Let's back up a moment to see how these trials work. Cell culture experiments, animal studies, and other human studies (often performed in other countries) form the basis for investigators to formulate a protocol, or plan, for the trial. The protocol determines how the trial will be organized, who will be entered, how the drugs will be administered, and how the results will be analyzed. It must be approved by the chief of the medical or surgical services involved and by administrators of the medical facility sponsoring the trial. Often the protocol is reviewed by experts familiar with the scientific studies initially supporting claims that the drug may be beneficial.

Statisticians then review the protocol to see whether statistically significant conclusions can be derived from the study. A major concern of statisticians is whether the number of subjects in the trial is large enough to give statistically significant results.

Finally, and perhaps most important, the human protection committee (also known as the human trials committee) reviews the plan and makes sure that the risk to patients is acceptable in view of possible benefits. This committee consists of both physicians and laypersons. The latter often look at the possible risks and benefits from the patient's point of view. One of the most important functions of the committee, besides approving trials, is helping to develop an informed consent form. This form tells patients clearly what risks and benefits they may expect from the trial therapy, and—without unduly frightening the patient—about side effects or other possible problems. (An example of an informed consent form appears in Appendix A.)

You should be able to get answers to any questions you have about a particular clinical trial from the investigator directing the study or from one of his or her associates. You can and should also read the protocol itself. However, this is technically difficult reading, and you may require assistance from the investigator or the clinical oncologist who is treating you. Without a doubt, you should also ask about the scientific studies that suggested in the first place that the trial drug(s) may be of benefit in treating cancer.

You should also be aware that at some time, either on entering the study or during it, patients are placed at random into different arms of the study and receive different treatments. This randomization of the patient into either the group receiving standard or no therapy (the "control" group) or into the group receiving the new drug (the "test" group) can be risky, since you cannot choose which group you are in. This procedure is necessary in order to evaluate a new therapy accurately. To achieve this, results of the trial drug are compared with standard therapy (the "control" group) or no therapy (the "placebo" group). In a properly controlled trial (called a double-blind study) no one knows—not the patients, not the investigator—which therapy is being given to which group of patients. This process, called blinding, eliminates psychological bias on the part of the investigator or the patient that may occur if treatment is identified. For example, a patient knowingly receiving standard therapy may assume it will not work; on the other hand, an investigator knowingly giving the new therapy may subjectively see improvement that is not actually present.

It is possible, therefore, that you will enter a clinical trial and not receive the new agent because you have not been randomly placed in one of these test groups. You should know, however, that if you do not respond to the given therapy, the protocol may allow switching you over to the test group. But no matter what happens, you have the right to leave the trial at any time and for any reason and revert back to standard treatment. Sometimes, however, the toxicity of the experimental therapy makes this difficult. The test drug may, for example, lower your blood counts, and you may not be able to receive standard therapy because it will lower these counts even more. Be sure to discuss these possibilities thoroughly with your doctor.

Clinical Trial Checklist

Here are some important questions you should discuss with your oncologist before entering a clinical trial.

- How likely am I to benefit from the new therapy?
- What alternatives to the new therapy do I have?
- How long will the trial and follow-up studies last?
- Will I need to be hospitalized? How long? How often?
- What side effects might occur?
- How are treatments given? (oral, IV, etc.)
- How often are treatments given?
- How long will each treatment take?
- Will blood tests be required to monitor therapy?
- Will other tests be necessary to evaluate the drug? (Sometimes tests are uncomfortable, and you should be aware of this possibility before starting therapy.)
- Where will testing be done? Home? Office? Clinic?
- How much of the cost will be paid by me? By my insurance company? By the government? By the drug company?

You most likely will have one or more sessions with the clinical oncologist and the physicians in charge of the study to address these concerns. You should feel free to discuss any questions for as long as you like, in as many sessions as you need, and until you feel that all your questions have been answered. Do not feel rushed into making a decision.

It's a good idea for you to research the study's sponsoring organization before making your final decision. You can determine if the organization is reputable by calling the Cancer Information Service hotline (1–800–4–CANCER), a program supported by the federal government and the National Institutes of Health (NIH). Currently active clinical trials are listed at this number. The information is reviewed by experts, and it is unlikely that disreputable trials would be included. Be aware of any trials that are not listed or are not sponsored by a hospital or cancer center. Also be sure to discuss the organization with your referring physician or oncologist.

Finally, be sure to discuss with your doctor the cost of trial drug administration, as well as any treatment needed to correct harmful results of the experimental therapy. Often government or drug company grants will pay all your costs once you have entered the trial, but in many cases at least some of the cost is borne by you, your family, or your insurance company. Insurance companies often refuse to pay for experimental therapies, however, so you should clearly understand beforehand who will pay for what. Ask your doctor to assist you with discussing this with the principal investigators in charge of the protocol, hospital administrators, or a representative of your insurance plan.

CHAPTER 4

Recovery Rates and Pain Control

Understanding Cancer Prognosis

In discussing prognosis, your oncologist uses many terms that you must understand in order to choose from alternative therapies. For this reason, and because the question of potential outcome is of great importance to you, let's survey the terms you will likely encounter when discussing prognosis and chemotherapy.

Survival and Cure Rates

A prognostication is a prediction of how a patient's disease is likely to progress with chemotherapy. It is based on both the results of clinical trials performed during the process of obtaining FDA approval and on the clinical experience with the drug after approval has been obtained. Of greatest interest to you is the cure rate expected after undergoing a course of chemotherapy. Cure rates are basically the same as survival rates, meaning the number of patients likely to have no evidence of disease remaining after a specific number of years. Evidence that the disease is still present is obtained by physical examination, X rays, and blood tests. For example, the cure rate for certain patients with Hodgkin's disease is 80 percent three years after treatment is stopped. This means that 80 percent of patients entering a study were alive and free of disease three years after their chemotherapy was completed. In the case of Hodgkin's disease, the vast majority of patients who relapse do so within two or three years after treatment, so this cure rate has been found to be relatively accurate.

Many cancer cure rates, however, are based on the percentage of patients entering a clinical trial who have no evidence of their cancer five years—rather than three—after starting treatment. Other patients, such as those with breast cancer, require ten years free of tumors before they are considered cured. Cure rates serve only as guidelines for evaluating how effective a treatment is. In individual patients, the disease may indeed recur even after the five- or ten-year NED (no evidence of disease) anniversary has passed.

Oncologists generally use survival rates. These rates specify only how many years have passed since therapy began. Rates published by the American Cancer Society are derived from cancer registries maintained by state and federal governments. The problem with the registries is that it is not always clear what therapy the patient did or did not get. Therefore, doctors obtain their information mainly from clinical trial data rather than the registries.

Doctors refer to survival rates when they report results of clinical trials and when they present options to their cancer patients. The doctor may tell a patient, for example, that 40 percent of patients are alive and free of disease five years after a certain type of chemotherapy began, while another 20 percent are alive, but with evidence of persistent or recurrent tumor. He or she might then compare this to the survival rates of patients treated with radiotherapy—instead of chemotherapy—in which only 20 percent are alive and free of disease at five years and 10 percent more are living, but with evidence of cancer.

To complicate matters, survival rates may be calculated in various ways: a direct method, a life table or actuarial method, or one based on sophisticated modeling techniques. These methods differ in the ways they account for dropouts from treatments, deaths from non-cancer-related causes, and adjustments for normal mortality rates. Do not be concerned with these details, but you should insist that the same methods of calculation are used for each treatment you are discussing or comparing. Keep in mind that in general it is very difficult for patients to understand how clinical trials are interpreted, and the details are best left to your oncologist.

Unfortunately, comparisons are complicated further by other factors, particularly if results from different clinical trials are being compared. The best comparisons are made when a trial uses large numbers of similar patients (usually conducted as a cooperative venture by several cancer centers) as the basis for choosing one therapy over another. Seldom is this possible, however, so it becomes important to look at the characteristics of the patients involved in the trials, i.e., the patient population, and at the design of the studies themselves.

Survival rates are based on clinical trials, each with its own set of unique factors that can affect the rates accordingly. The following checklist may be helpful in discussing a clinical trial and the resulting survival rate with your oncologist.

At what stage of disease were the patients when the study began?

The most important consideration when looking at the patient population in a study is how far the cancer had spread before treatment started. Was the disease localized, or had it spread to nearby organs or to distant sites? The extent of spread or the stage of the disease must be the same in all patients in order to make a valid comparison between therapies given to different patient groups or between different clinical trials. For example, patients with breast cancer confined to the breast (early stage) are likely to do better with a given therapy than patients whose breast cancer has spread to other organs such as the lung, liver, and brain (late stage).

*Was there a control group? If so, what treatment (if any) did
patients in the group receive?*

The trial used for comparison should include a control group, i.e.,
patients who receive standard therapy (or no treatment) rather than
the experimental chemotherapy. Without a control group, there is
no scientific way to compare study results. Because cancers progress
at their own natural pace, investigators must separate the progress
of the disease from the effect of chemotherapy. The only way to
do this is to follow some patients with the experimental therapy
and others without it. For ethical reasons, however, all patients in
the trial may receive some sort of treatment. Therefore, instead of
receiving no treatment at all, the control group may receive a standard, but perhaps ineffective, treatment and the experimental
group will receive the therapy being tested.

How many patients were in each control and experimental group?

Enough patients should be included in both control and experimental groups to enable a valid statistical comparison. A certain
number of patients must be in each group in order to compute
valid statistical probabilities that indicate whether the experimental
therapy is superior to control therapy or no therapy. Generally at
least twenty patients in each group (and sometimes many more)
are needed before statisticians can tell us if the experimental therapy is an improvement in terms of survival, quality of life, or side
effects. The number of patients needed depends on many factors,
but one of the most important is how effective the experimental
drug is. To show small improvements in survival or quality of life,
large groups may be needed. A very effective drug, on the other
hand, may need only a relatively few patients in each group in
order to prove that the therapy is beneficial. In fact, if the statisticians see that the experimental group is doing better, they may
interrupt the study, saying that it is not ethical to deny the experimental therapy to patients in the control group.

How long were patients followed and results measured?

Patients should be followed and results measured over a period of time long enough to justify concluding that the experimental treatment actually changed (or did not change) the course of the disease. An acceptable time period may be ten years for some tumors yet only two years for others. The experimental group may improve at first, but, when patients are followed over a period of months or years after therapy, it may become clear that the benefit is not as great as it had seemed. The experimental therapy may not affect quality of life or survival, and the long-term side effects may be too severe to justify use of the new program. If benefit is not seen soon (within weeks or a few months), continued treatment probably is not justified.

How many patients dropped out before participating in follow-up testing? Were statistical methods appropriate?

It is important to know if there were only a few patients who did not participate in follow-up testing and if appropriate methods were used for statistical calculation and comparisons. Statistical analysis has many pitfalls. If too many patients drop out or change therapy, the conclusions from statistical computations may be affected, so that it becomes impossible to interpret results. The choice of statistical methods to analyze data is very difficult, and the use of inappropriate methods can lead to false conclusions regarding the effectiveness and safety of chemotherapy drugs.

Most cancer patients do not have enough information to evaluate the results of clinical trials. They depend on their oncologist or primary physician to make this evaluation and explain relative risks to them in an understandable manner. For some patients, their education and background will allow detailed discussion of the underlying information on which the oncologist's recommendations are based. For many others, a detailed discussion is not possible and may only add to the patient's confusion and anxiety. You, however, should ask your doctor any questions you feel are necessary to completely understand your treatment options. Use care in selecting a doctor to perform this analysis and to help you use the information in making your own treatment decisions (see Chapter 1).

Frequently, the differences between types of cancer therapy are seen only when comparisons are made between responders—patients whose tumor size decreases—and nonresponders, those whose tumor size decreases only slightly or not at all, or whose disease actually gets worse. In this type of study all patients receive the same test therapy. This is a distinctly different comparison from one between patients receiving an experimental treatment and those getting standard therapy. When only responders vs. nonresponders are compared, no valid conclusions regarding effectiveness can be made. Although responders may appear to survive longer, this difference may be unrelated to the effectiveness of the treatment. For example, more nonresponders may have succumbed to toxic effects of the treatment they received, causing an apparent advantage in survival time of responders compared to nonresponders. Your oncologist should be well aware of this problem and should not use data based on comparisons of responders and nonresponders in recommending therapy. For these reasons, fewer of these comparisons are now published in medical literature than in the past. If your physician talks about this type of study, instead of controlled studies, you should ask if other studies have actually compared control groups with experimental groups, as described above. Keep in mind that reported benefits of an experimental therapy are reliable only if properly designed studies have shown that the treatment is effective.

Quality of Life

Although survival and cure rates are most important to patients, other considerations may go into a decision to accept chemotherapy. With many cancers, the cure rate, particularly when the cancer has spread, is very low and survival is short. In these cases, a patient's quality of life becomes an issue. Will the therapy allow the patient to carry on normal, everyday activities? Clinical trial results may show whether or not patients have a better quality of life after a particular chemotherapy. Can patients take better care of themselves? Do they need less assistance? Are they less disabled and able to leave the hospital? One way physicians look at this issue is to use the Karnofsky Performance Status scale, which allows points in each of these activities to measure the effect of chemotherapy on quality of life. Alleviation of pain, improved nutritional status, relief from bleeding or infection, and improved mood are other quality of life issues. The possibility of improvement in any of these areas can influence patients to accept chemotherapy even when there is little hope for improvement in survival or cure rate.

Many clinical trials report not only the number of patients who completely respond to therapy and have no evidence of residual cancer, but also the number of patients who have a partial response. This could mean that there has been some shrinkage of the tumor, improvement in quality of life, or better pain control. Unfortunately, partial responses do not generally mean improved survival and are of use only when considering quality of life issues rather than a cure. These considerations are closely related to the dual role of chemotherapy. First, it is hoped that such therapy will cure the disease. But in many cases chemotherapy plays a second role, that of palliation, which will only improve the patient's immediate condition or temporarily control symptoms. Your physician should explain early in the course of treatment whether the goal is to cure the disease or to palliate your symptoms. If he or she does not, ask. Too many patients assume that their chemotherapy will cure or prolong survival when doctors know it will only help control pain and suffering.

Side Effects

Second only to survival in the patient's mind are the side effects or toxicity of the drug. In every clinical trial, observed side effects, such as vomiting, hair loss, or infection, must be reported, along with an estimate of their frequency and severity. Oncologists are morally obligated and legally responsible to inform you of the risks associated with the proposed chemotherapy. Most chemotherapy complications are treatable, and you should be assured that your physician will provide such therapy if it is necessary. Many patients have great difficulty in hearing about or understanding the risks of chemotherapy. Sometimes the patient's age, education, temperament, or other factors interfere. Have your family members participate in your discussions of risks with your doctor, especially if there is something you do not understand. Then you and your family can review at home the material presented by your physician, get answers to your questions directly, or telephone your oncologist for more information as questions come up.

Here are some questions you should ask about side effects when considering a particular type of chemotherapy:

- What are the side effects? Which are likely to occur?
- How often do they occur?
- Are they severe enough to interfere with work or activities of daily living?
- Are there ways to avoid or reduce the side effects?
- Do therapies that reduce side effects have side effects of their own? For example, will drugs taken to control vomiting make me drowsy, interfering with my ability to drive or work?
- Whom do I contact for help with side effects? Are oncology nurses available for this sort of help?

Pre-Approval Drugs

If you are scheduled to receive chemotherapy not approved by the FDA, you will be required to sign a form stating that you have been informed of potential side effects and understand the risks of the procedure. Before the treatment begins, it is especially important for you and your family to know the prognosis—the chance of being cured, or, at least, the odds of improving your quality of life, as well as potential side effects and financial costs of the drug. Until recently, drugs not yet approved by the FDA were supplied free, since they were experimental. However, the law has been changed; drug companies can now charge for drugs that are non-

FDA approved but are likely to be approved soon. Some manufacturers do, therefore, charge for experimental drugs, while others do not. Be sure to confirm this with your oncologist before proceeding.

Alternative Treatments

Oncologists can usually forecast the course that the cancer will take. The difficult part is forecasting the rate of the cancer's progress. Many times, physicians are amazed at how fast or how slowly the cancer spreads. Sometimes death comes sooner and at other times much later than expected. When discussing prognosis, therefore, you should always ask about alternative treatments. This is particularly true with cancers that are not curable, are unlikely to respond completely, or can be treated only with toxic drugs. Unfortunately, the most common types of cancer fall into one or more of these categories.

At some point you will probably ask: What will happen if I decide not to accept chemotherapy? What treatments other than chemotherapy are available to me? If you decide not to receive chemotherapy, your only option is to let the cancer take its course while you consider three alternative therapies intended to palliate your symptoms and maintain your quality of life:

1. Pain-killing drugs or other methods for pain relief (see below) along with symptomatic therapy, such as medication for vomiting.
2. Transfusion of blood or blood products for anemia or bleeding (see Chapter 8).
3. Radiation of affected areas to reduce pain and other symptoms (see Chapter 8).

If you decide not to accept chemotherapy, discuss these alternatives with your physician. He or she will arrange for treatments and medications appropriate to your situation.

Pain Control

Cancer chemotherapy palliates many patients, relieving their pain and other discomforts (see Chapter 6). But for some, pain relief does not last; for others, chemotherapy is not available or does not help. Patients often fear uncontrollable pain more than the cancer itself. When pain-free, they can usually forget, at least for a time, that they have cancer. With modern drugs, there is no reason for patients with cancer to suffer pain. What follows is an approach to cancer pain that has proven effective over the years. Many other approaches exist and may have advantages, but the one presented here is effective and is used by a great many oncologists.

While considering the use of pain-relieving drugs, the physician must search for and treat—with radiation, surgery, or cancer chemotherapy—any cause of pain for which a remedy is possible. For example, bone pain can be relieved with radiation therapy given over a short period of time, often with few side effects. Relief occurs within a few days or weeks and is often long-lasting. Pain caused by tumors entering or pressing on nerves may also respond to radiation therapy. Obstruction of the bowel or ducts that drain organs such as the pancreas, bladder, or liver can be relieved, and the associated pain decreased, by radiation therapy or surgery intended to bypass the obstruction. Infections, such as painful abscesses, which result in swelling or accumulation of fluids in closed body spaces, are relieved with surgical drainage or antibiotics. Radiation helps patients with obstructed drainage in the lymphatic system or blood circulation. This approach often succeeds in patients with lymph node diseases in which drainage is blocked by malignant cells, or in patients with blockage of large veins in the abdomen, causing fluid to accumulate in the abdomen and legs. If you are experiencing any of these types of pain, ask your doctor about these treatments.

Chemotherapy itself can cause pain, requiring reduced dosage or elimination of certain drugs from the therapy. For example, vincristine causes pain by some unknown effect on the nerves. The pain usually occurs in the feet, hands, or jaw. Because nerves are affected, the pain has a burning, tingling, or shooting quality and is often intermittent rather than constant. Many patients have painful inflammation and ulcers in the mouth (mucositis) after chemotherapy begins. Bleeding or infection caused by chemotherapy is often quite painful, especially if the brain, abdominal organs, or muscles are involved.

Another painful complication is shingles, an infection caused by the *herpes zoster* virus. Painful skin blisters appear almost anywhere on the skin, often heralded by unexplained burning or sharp pains on one side or in one part of the body. The pain can persist even after the blisters have healed. New antiviral antibiotics show some promise in relieving pain and preventing the rash from spreading. Sometimes a short course of cortisonelike drugs is given to relieve this condition.

Drugs called analgesics are the mainstay for treatment of cancer pain. Despite surgery, radiation, and chemotherapy, most cancer victims will experience pain that can be relieved only by these agents. Mild to moderate pain usually responds to either aspirin (650 to 1,000 milligrams, equal to two or three regular-strength tablets) or acetaminophen (1,000 milligrams, equal to two extra-strength tablets). Acetaminophen has one advantage over aspirin: it does not cause stomach bleeding or irritation in some patients as aspirin can. Also, patients with low platelet counts because of their cancer or chemotherapy cannot use aspirin for fear of its causing bleeding into vital organs. Combining aspirin or acetaminophen with other analgesics enhances pain relief and makes it last longer. Other drugs with similar potency but more side effects are codeine, pentazocine, and propoxyphene. Mental confusion and constipation are commonly encountered with these drugs.

A new class of analgesics, called NSAIDs (nonsteroidal, anti-inflammatory drugs), has helped patients with moderate cancer pain. Although similar in action to aspirin, they appear to be more effective than aspirin or acetaminophen, especially when used in combination with narcotics. Stomach upset occurs but can be helped by taking the drugs with meals, antacids, or with a drug called sucrafate. Sucrafate relieves stomach irritation in patients who cannot normally tolerate NSAIDs even when given with meals or antacids. The NSAIDs, such as ibuprofen, diflunisal, or naproxen, can be used alone for mild to moderate pain or in combination with narcotics. When NSAIDs are combined with narcotics such as codeine or methadone, lower dosages of narcotics are required to control more severe pain. NSAIDs do increase slightly the risk of bleeding in patients with platelet counts lowered by chemotherapy or radiotherapy. If you use these drugs you must, therefore, report to your oncologist any signs of bleeding, such as black-and-blue marks, nosebleeds, or bleeding gums.

Psychological Techniques

Attitude and behavior can be extremely important in relieving mild to moderate pain. This theory is based on observation rather than scientific research. This approach seems to depend mostly on the patient's outlook: those who maintain their optimism can control pain to a surprising degree. It is important that your oncologist keeps you informed about the goals of chemotherapy. Most patients find it is best to maintain a mixture of hope and realistic expectation. Many do this by keeping a diary of events and their reactions to help lower fear and anxiety, two emotions that accentuate pain. As bad as cancer may be, some patients often fantasize that the situation is even worse than it is likely to be. An informed patient, however, is more relaxed and in less pain than one who is not. Reassurances from your oncologist that any pain will be treated, with narcotics if necessary, is an important part of the doctor-patient relationship. You may also find it helpful to keep a list of questions to ask your physician or nurse on a regular basis. Getting answers to your questions will help relieve your fear and anxiety, and thereby reduce your pain.

Distraction is an excellent way to relieve pain. Stay active with your work or hobbies and keep in touch with your friends, relatives, and other cancer patients. Patient support groups (see Appendix B) are usually available in urban areas and are excellent sources of information and emotional support, especially for patients who have been recently diagnosed. These groups may have a negative aspect if you become attached to a fellow cancer patient who dies.

Also, some group members might focus too much on their cancer and ignore their potentially supportive families and friends. Exercise, such as walking, swimming, jogging, or aerobics, can be of great help too, especially if you have previously used exercise to relieve stress and tension.

Relaxation techniques not only help with pain but may relieve side effects such as nausea and vomiting. Find a quiet moment and place. Think of a pleasant scene, stare at a blank wall, concentrate on slow rhythmic breathing, or repeatedly chant a number or a word. All these techniques work to relieve pain. Control of pain and relief of anxiety can be obtained by using biofeedback to produce a relaxed state of mind and body. Biofeedback uses special machines to monitor a patient's brain waves and thereby help control heart rate, blood pressure, and muscle tension. Self-hypnosis has also been suggested to control discomfort, but it usually relieves only mild pain. Check with your oncology clinic for instructions in these relaxation techniques.

A behavioral technique called imagery is similar to other relaxation techniques, except that it uses *all* the senses. The National Cancer Institute's booklet *Chemotherapy and You* describes this method of using imagery to relieve discomfort:

Concentrate on breathing comfortably from your abdomen. Imagine a ball of healing energy, perhaps a white light, forming somewhere in your body. When you can see the ball of energy, imagine that the air you breathe in blows it to any part of the body where you feel pain or discomfort such as nausea. When you breathe out, picture the air moving the ball away from the body, taking with it the pain or discomfort and tension. (Be careful not to blow as you breathe out; breathe naturally.) Continue to picture the ball moving toward you and away each time you breathe in or out. You may see the ball getting bigger as it takes more and more discomfort and tension away. To end the imagery, count slowly to three, breathe in deeply, open your eyes, and say to yourself, "I feel alert and relaxed." Begin moving about slowly.

Acupuncture and TENS

Acupuncture has helped some patients, but it is expensive and it loses effectiveness over time and as pain becomes more severe. Trained acupuncturists insert sterilized needles into pain-relieving sites on the skin and, in some cases, deliver a small amount of electricity through the needle and into the skin. For reasons that are unknown, this age-old technique relieves pain.

For control of mild to moderate pain, a small electric pulse generator has been developed that delivers electrical impulses to painful parts of the body. Electrodes are pasted to the skin at points corresponding to sites acupuncturists use to control pain. These devices, called TENS (transcutaneous electrical nerve stimulation) units, are worth a try if pain is not too severe and is localized within a small area. The units may be purchased or rented and are often paid for by medical insurance plans. The device can be activated by the patient when pain is present. Side effects are negligible. On the downside, however, pain control may not be complete, and only one or two areas can be treated at any one time. Pain relief often diminishes over time. As pain increases and the treatment's effectiveness lessens, you should discuss with your doctor the next options in pain control, such as narcotics.

Narcotics

The drugs and techniques described above are first-line resources in dealing with pain. Narcotics, such as morphine, methadone, oxycodone, or codeine, represent the second line of defense against moderate to severe pain. These drugs are given orally with a full dose of acetaminophen. For temporary pain, physicians usually administer as-needed doses of a combination drug such as oxycodone plus acetaminophen (Percocet) or codeine plus acetaminophen. To combat chronic pain, however, doctors may resort to something stronger such as methadone or morphine with full doses of acetaminophen or NSAIDs. Doctors divide doses of narcotics throughout the day and even at night. Your doctor may, however, prescribe long-acting morphine preparations that need to be taken by mouth only two or three times in twenty-four hours. Examples include MS-Contin (morphine sulfate controlled release) or Roxanol (morphine sulfate concentrated oral solution). Hydromorphone is another powerful narcotic that is also available as a rectal suppository, tablet, or injection. A suppository has its advantages, because it assures that the drug will stay in a patient's system even if he or she is vomiting. This drug is also available as a liquid for patients who cannot swallow tablets. Always be aware that one major problem is overdosing, because these drugs have a tendency to accumulate in the body. Confusion, agitation, sedation, breathing difficulty, and other major effects on the brain limit how much the patient can take and still function. Side effects include constipation, nausea, and vomiting. Constipation can be relieved by stool softeners, liquids, and cathartics such as milk of magnesia or lactulose. Nausea and vomiting are generally helped by antinauseants such as Compazine (perchlorperazine). Trials of various combinations of analgesics, some not mentioned here, may benefit individual patients, and with trial and error, all cancer patients can be relieved of pain.

In the past, two issues surrounding the use of narcotics in cancer patients have caused concern. First, there was concern about addiction. Cancer patients rarely become addicted, however, and, in fact, most are anxious to get off these drugs. In the terminally ill patient, worry about addiction is obviously secondary to pain relief. A second issue of concern was undermedication. Physicians were reluctant to prescribe doses high enough to relieve the pain, for fear of addicting the patient and perhaps opening themselves up to criticism by their peers or the public. Today, this concern has been resolved, and there is no social or legal reason why cancer patients cannot receive doses of narcotics adequate for their needs.

If a patient is incurably ill and cancer has spread throughout the body, the pain may be so severe that it no longer responds to oral medications. Yet injections into the muscles may be too painful if the patient has lost a lot of weight and lacks skin and muscle tissue.

These intramuscular injections may also cause bleeding into the puncture sites. Intravenous morphine, therefore, is by far the best medication for severe pain. If high enough doses are used, continuous intravenous infusion (morphine drip) will control almost any pain. The patient will become heavily sedated and should be unaware of any physical or mental discomfort. The mood-elevating effect of intravenous morphine is also beneficial to some patients. Often the patient has a degree of limited function, especially if cared for at home. Various devices have been developed to allow patients to self-administer a dose of intravenous morphine whenever they need it. These devices, however, are still experimental and may not be available everywhere.

For a small number of patients with severe pain, intravenous narcotic drugs are unacceptable because they oversedate, cause mental confusion, or otherwise leave patients unable to function. Their pain is too severe, however, to be relieved by acetaminophen or NSAIDs. To help such patients, neurosurgeons and anesthesiologists have developed a number of procedures. Nerves that transmit pain signals can be surgically cut, relieving pain for some of these patients. However, the patient may lose function in the arms or legs, and only one side of the body can be treated in this way. Alternatively, narcotics or novocainelike drugs may be injected into the area surrounding the spinal column. These epidural blocks substantially relieve pain, but again at a cost. For example, daily injections of morphine, through a catheter into the lower spinal column, may make breathing difficult. In a similar technique, alcohol or phenol is injected, giving good results with little danger of breathing problems. Because the alcohol or phenol needs to be given only every few months, this type of treatment does not require placing a permanent catheter. Needless to say, patients do not look forward to any of these procedures, but they can bring welcome relief from pain in some situations.

Antidepressants, such as amitriptyline, also enhance pain control for some patients. In addition to the usual analgesics, these drugs are given as a single dose at bedtime. Only some patients benefit; others cannot tolerate side effects, often characterized by patients as a spacey feeling. Antihistamines and cortisonelike drugs, called adrenal corticosteroids, such as prednisone or Decadron (dexamethasone), also add to the beneficial effects of narcotic analgesics.

Ask your oncologist for the latest information about pain control techniques. Although there have been few advances in pain control in recent years, oncologists track this area very closely.

CHAPTER 5

Chemotherapy
That Works Well

Few cancers are curable with chemotherapy alone. Those that are include Hodgkin's disease, certain forms of non-Hodgkin's lymphoma, acute leukemia, testicular cancer, and cancer of the fetal placenta. Other malignancies, including other types of non-Hodgkin's lymphoma, myeloma, and breast cancer, are not curable with chemotherapy alone, but symptoms can be significantly controlled for years by successful chemotherapy.

Breast Cancer

Patients with breast cancer are usually treated by medical oncologists, who are trained to diagnose and treat all malignancies. Sometimes, however, they are treated by oncologists trained in gynecology or other specialties. As with most other cancers, surgery, radiation therapy, and chemotherapy are the primary treatments for cure and for palliation (symptom relief) of breast cancer. This type of cancer is not curable by chemotherapy alone, but with surgery some otherwise incurable patients can be cured. More often, however, chemotherapy is used to relieve symptoms of breast cancer, and good results are often possible for many years.

Male breast cancer is rare; nevertheless, treatment is similar to that used for female breast cancer. Surgical removal and radiotherapy are used to treat the primary breast tumor. Since growth of the tumor in men depends on the male hormone, androgen, some patients benefit from the removal of the testicles to decrease production of that hormone. Large doses of estrogens, female hormones, may also relieve symptoms. When these therapies fail, chemotherapy with the same agents and drug combinations as used in female patients may help control symptoms.

Early Breast Cancer

Treatment of breast cancer is very controversial. Theories about the most effective strategies to use are constantly changing and adjusting according to the availability of new information and research. Be aware that treatment guidelines presented here may not reflect the best course of therapy for you, so be sure to discuss these options with your doctor.

Almost all cancers confined to the breast itself and measuring less than one inch are curable with surgery and radiotherapy. In these cases, chemotherapy is usually not needed. However, if the tumor is larger than one inch or if the disease has spread to the axillary lymph glands on the side where the tumor is located, chemotherapy is likely to be a significant part of treatment. Lymph is a fluid that functions in the lymphatic system in a way resembling the blood in the circulatory system. Lymph flows through lymphatic vessels, mopping up waste material that accumulates during various biological processes. Lymph glands, also called lymph nodes, are located throughout the body to filter the waste from the lymph much like the way the spleen and liver filter waste from the blood. Axillary lymph glands, located in the axilla (armpit), filter lymph fluid draining from the breast. Cancer cells from the breast may grow in these nodes and may also spread widely to other parts of the body. Lymph nodes affected by the cancer are considered local metastases, and the sites to which the cancer spreads are called distant metastases.

Additive (adjuvant) chemotherapy. In the case of local metastases, chemotherapy can add to the effects of surgery and radiation used during the initial treatment. This additive, or adjuvant, chemotherapy destroys cancer cells that may be present elsewhere in the body even in early stages of the disease. Chemotherapy can, in this case, help cure early breast cancer. In contrast, patients with advanced breast tumors can hope only to relieve symptoms with palliative chemotherapy. The following histories of two typical patients illustrate the difference between additive and palliative chemotherapy:

At the age of thirty-nine, Mrs. R. discovered a small lump in her right breast. A mammogram indicated a tumor and, later, a biopsy revealed a definite malignancy. She chose to have her breast removed by an operation called a modified radical mastectomy. Her breast and underlying tissues (including muscles of her chest wall) and the lymph glands in her right armpit were removed and examined by the pathologist. Mrs. R.'s lymph glands showed cancer in three of the nodes. Because she was premenopausal, her physician recommended additive chemotherapy. She received a combination of three drugs given in monthly cycles for a total of six months. Now, six years later, there has been no recurrence of cancer.

Mrs. B., at the age of sixty-five, discovered a lump in her right breast which, on biopsy, proved to be malignant. Ten lymph nodes removed from her right armpit were positive for cancer. No additive chemotherapy was given, but the patient was treated with tamoxifen, a drug resembling the female hormone, estrogen. Three years later, she developed pains in her bones and abdomen. Testing revealed spread of her cancer to the liver and bones. Her doctors began palliative chemotherapy to relieve her symptoms and continued the treatments for one year. During this time, she was free of pain, but cancer was evident on her X rays. Her disease has now become more painful and, despite chemotherapy with several different drugs, her condition continues to deteriorate.

The treatment of early breast cancer with additive chemotherapy is complex. Oncologists must consider all the factors, such as the size of the tumor, whether or not the axillary lymph nodes are affected, the patient's menopausal status, and the results of the estrogen receptor assay (explained below) done on the breast tissue obtained during the initial surgery. Treatment recommendations are constantly being changed by the National Cancer Institutes and other research organizations. Also, oncologists may differ in their interpretation of the studies upon which recommendations are based.

As I just illustrated, the menopausal status and the stage of the breast cancer play important roles in determining a patient's treatment options. Premenopausal women have not yet stopped having menstrual periods; perimenopausal women have not menstruated for up to three years; and postmenopausal women have not menstruated for three years or more.

Premenopausal patients. Premenopausal patients whose disease is present in only one breast and axillary lymph nodes (on the same side as the tumor) are almost always offered additive chemotherapy. Recently, premenopausal patients without lymph node involvement have also been advised to undergo additive chemotherapy. Two to five drugs are given over a period of about six months. Women are about 15 to 20 percent more likely to survive, free of disease, for five or more years if they receive this additive chemotherapy than if they do not. Premenopausal patients with more than four cancerous axillary lymph nodes are at high risk for spread of the cancer to other parts of the body. For this group, researchers are testing new and aggressive chemotherapy programs that use more drugs at higher dosages.

Talk with your oncologist about treatment dosage, but remember that most experts agree that full doses of chemotherapy given as scheduled are necessary for additive chemotherapy to be beneficial. Physicians who reduce doses because they fear that the patient will be made sick are probably compromising the final outcome of ther-

apy. Any attempt to use lower or less frequent drug doses will
reduce chances of survival. One expert has said that a 20 percent
reduction in scheduled drug dosage can decrease chances of survival by as much as 50 percent. He adds that tens of thousands of
women will relapse unless full doses are administered.

Postmenopausal patients. Postmenopausal women, on the other
hand, do not always benefit from additive chemotherapy, regardless of how many lymph nodes are affected. Doctors agree, however, that an additive hormonal therapy, usually with tamoxifen,
as I will explain later, improves survival in postmenopausal women
who have cancerous breast lumps and positive lymph nodes but no
evidence of spread to other organs. This type of hormone therapy
is also ideal for additive therapy in postmenopausal women who
have negative nodes. Clinical studies have shown that these hormone treatments delay the recurrence of breast cancer in postmenopausal women in a way similar to that of premenopausal
women who are treated with additive chemotherapy.

Estrogen receptor assay. To determine if a patient is a strong
candidate for hormone therapy, doctors perform what is called an
estrogen receptor assay. This is a biochemical test done on breast
cancer cells removed during surgery. It looks for structures called
receptors on tumor cell walls that bind the female hormone, estrogen. Tumors bearing these receptors are much more likely to
be susceptible to the cancer-killing effects of hormones or hor-
monelike drugs such as tamoxifen. Most postmenopausal women
have estrogen receptors on their cancer cells. The few who do not
probably will not benefit from tamoxifen and will generally be
treated with standard chemotherapy. For most postmenopausal
women, tamoxifen will, at least, delay the tumor from recurring.
This drug has few side effects, but it is expensive. The manufacturer (Stuart Pharmaceuticals) will supply free tablets to patients
in financial need. A few patients receiving tamoxifen, particularly
those whose tumors have spread to the bones, will develop increased levels of calcium in their blood. Because this can be dangerous, blood tests are needed when treatment begins. Overall,
tamoxifen has fewer side effects than chemotherapy, and the survival benefits are similar.

Hormone therapy in general is sometimes confused with chemotherapy, because hormones are chemicals, too. Tamoxifen works
by mimicking the biochemical effects of estrogens on breast cancer
cells. In an as yet unknown way, these effects slow the growth of
breast cancer cells. Progesterone is yet another type of hormone
that may relieve symptoms for patients who initially respond to
tamoxifen, but then relapse. Hormones are preferable to chemotherapeutic agents because they have fewer side effects and their
benefits are often longer-lasting.

Additive Chemotherapy Program
for Early Breast Cancer Patients

Additive or adjuvant chemotherapy (intended to cure) for early
breast cancer usually includes some combination of four drugs:
cyclophosphamide, methotrexate, adriamycin, and 5-fluorouracil.
A commonly used program, called CMF, employs cyclophosphamide, relatively small doses of methotrexate, and 5-fluorouracil,
given every three or four weeks for six months. It is important that
your doctor administers full doses and strictly follows the therapeutic schedule. This program is more or less considered the standard against which all others are judged. Its main advantages are
that it is easy to administer, relatively free from side effects, and
adds 10 to 20 percent to the long-term survival rate, which is about
50 percent without chemotherapy and 60 to 70 percent with chemotherapy.

Other programs add adriamycin or use large doses of methotrexate. These programs, called CAMF and super-CMF, respec-
tively, are usually administered during four- to six-week cycles. The
super-CMF program requires an antidote ("leucovorin rescue") to
counter the toxic effects of larger doses of methotrexate (see Chapter 8). Because the antidote must be given at precise times and
because special precautions are necessary to prevent kidney damage
from methotrexate, patients who receive these programs must de-
vote a great deal of time and effort to their therapy. Although some
oncologists believe that this intensive therapy is better than CMF
alone, increased effectiveness in prolonging survival rates has not

yet been proven. (The side effects patients may have in these programs are described in Chapter 7.)

Inflammatory breast cancer. Chemotherapy has also helped patients with inflammatory breast cancer, a rare tumor previously thought to be untreatable. The tumor has a distinctive appearance under the microscope, and it may appear as spreading ulcers on the chest wall. Patients experience severe edema (fluid accumulation) in the affected breast and surrounding skin. For this highly malignant and often fast-growing tumor, combination therapy with tamoxifen, together with multiple drug chemotherapy, always including adriamycin, often yields a near-complete and sometimes long-lasting remission.

Hodgkin's Disease and Non-Hodgkin's Lymphomas

The first malignant disease successfully treated with chemotherapy was lymphoma. To understand how chemotherapy is used in lymphoma, we must first understand the origin of the cells—called lymphocytes—that become malignant in these diseases.

Lymphocytes

Various types of cells circulate within our blood. One of these cells, the lymphocyte, provides one mechanism for defending the body against infection. The defense mechanism itself is called the immune response, and the cells and organs involved make up the immune system. There are two types of immune response: (1) immunity provided by the cells themselves, that is, their ability to directly destroy foreign bacteria or cells; and (2) immunity provided by the production of substances called antibodies. Antibodies are proteins made by lymphocytes, which prepare foreign materials for destruction by other lymphocytes or related cells. Should these lymphocytes become malignant, diseases such as malignant lymphomas and lymphocytic leukemias develop.

Lymphocytes arise in two organs of the human body: (1) the

bone marrow, located in spaces inside the ribs, breastbone, spine, and pelvic (hip) bones; and (2) in the thymus, a small gland inside the chest cavity behind the breastbone. Lymphocytes migrate to all parts of the body and are found not only in the blood but also in structures such as lymph nodes. These are the same lymph nodes, or lymph glands, that swell and become painful during viral illness, such as colds or sore throats. Every part of the human body has either lymph nodes or collections of lymphocytes, which fight infection and participate in the immune response to foreign agents or tumor cells.

No one knows for certain how lymphocytes become malignant. Probably several factors interact to transform normally helpful lymphocytes into malignant cells that destroy healthy tissues and ultimately kill their host. Viruses, such as the Epstein-Barr (EB) virus that causes the benign disease called infectious mononucleosis, have been implicated as causes of malignant lymphomas. So, where chemotherapy is now our only hope of curing some patients with these diseases, it may be possible in the future to employ antiviral vaccines to prevent lymphomas from developing.

Lymphoma Diagnosis

Patients with lymphoma may initially visit a doctor because they have symptoms that include unexplained fevers; lumps that prove to be enlarged lymph nodes; an enlarged spleen, an organ in the upper left side of the abdomen; unexplained weight loss; or drenching night sweats.

To diagnose lymphoma, it is necessary to obtain a biopsy; that is, a sample of lymph node tissue is removed for examination by a pathologist, a physician who specializes in diagnosing biopsies. The pathologist can separate malignant lymphomas into two categories. The first, Hodgkin's disease, involves destruction of the normal structure of the patient's lymph glands by abnormal cells including a very unusual one, called the Reed-Sternberg cell. When Reed-Sternberg cells are present in a lymph node, the pathologist returns the diagnosis of Hodgkin's disease. This information, along with the extent to which the disease has spread in the body, de-

termines the type of chemotherapy or other treatment most likely
to help the patient. The other type of lymphoma is called non-
Hodgkin's lymphoma and requires somewhat different chemotherapy.

Lymphoma Therapy

As mentioned, therapy for lymphoma is determined by its type
and by how much it has spread throughout the body. Therefore,
lymphoma patients are subjected to a whole battery of tests, X rays,
scans, and sometimes even surgical exploration of the abdomen or
other body cavities, in order to find out how far the disease has
progressed.

Unlike other cancers, surgery plays no role in the treatment of
lymphoma, although, as mentioned, surgery is extremely important
for diagnosis and sometimes for determining how far the disease
has spread. Generally, if the lymphoma involves lymph nodes in
only a very few areas, X ray treatments can cure the disease. This
is particularly true with Hodgkin's disease involving only the neck
and axillary (underarm) nodes.

When lymphoma spreads into lymph nodes throughout the body
or actually invades other organs such as the liver or lung (something
that happens frequently with non-Hodgkin's lymphoma), chemotherapy may cure or at least relieve symptoms. Although the principles of treatment are similar for both Hodgkin's disease and
non-Hodgkin's lymphomas, there is an important difference, especially in the expected outcome.

Treatment of Hodgkin's Disease

All four subtypes of Hodgkin's disease—lymphocytic predomi-
nant, mixed cellularity, nodular sclerosis, and lymphocytic deple-
tion—are treated similarly and with the intention to cure. Doctors
prescribe six or more courses of MOPP (mustargen, Oncovin, procarbazine, and prednisone), ABVD (adriamycin, bleomycin, vinblastine, and DTIC) or, by alternating treatments, use both
programs. Some alternative programs are also available, but MOPP

and ABVD are standard therapy. In Chapter 2, I listed the typical chemotherapy combinations for Hodgkin's disease. Side effects common to each of these programs include the usual nausea, vomiting hours after intravenous infusions, hair loss, and increased risk of infection and bleeding.

The MOPP program has been available for many years, and only one other program has a better overall cure rate. However, a large percentage of patients who use this program become permanently infertile and a few develop acute leukemias and other malignancies later in life after the Hodgkin's disease is cured. Hormone treatments can sometimes prevent infertility in females; nevertheless, if you wish to avoid infertility, for whatever reason, find another equally effective program. Ask your doctor about ABVD. It has a cure rate somewhat better than MOPP, seems to preserve fertility, and to date has not caused as many secondary malignancies as MOPP has. There is a drawback, however. More commonly associated with ABVD than with MOPP are heart complications related to the use of adriamycin, and severe vomiting from the DTIC it includes. It remains to be seen whether ABVD will be an overall improvement over MOPP. Recently, oncologists have attempted to decrease side effects and improve the cure rate by treating Hodgkin's patients with alternating cycles of ABVD and MOPP. Although this approach appears sound, no long-term scientific studies have yet proven that this program is better than ABVD or MOPP alone.

Chemotherapy plus radiotherapy. Patients sometimes receive radiotherapy after chemotherapy if lymph nodes in a particular area, such as the abdomen, are greatly enlarged at the time of diagnosis. Radiotherapists recommend this treatment based on the fact that, if relapse occurs, it often appears in areas where lymph nodes are enlarged. However, no one has shown that this radiotherapy actually increases the patient's survival time. In certain advanced cases of Hodgkin's disease, the oncologist will prescribe radiotherapy interspersed between cycles of chemotherapy. Statistics show that more patients have complete remission, that is, they are rendered free of detectable disease, if both chemotherapy and radiotherapy are used. Unhappily, however, these patients also seem to develop a larger than expected number—though still a small percentage— of secondary malignancies, so that is has become very difficult for doctors to advise their patients about this combination of therapies. Many oncologists claim that the improved survival rate benefits more patients, thereby outweighing the much smaller number that are afflicted with a second cancer. Only further observation of patients treated with different programs will finally answer this very difficult, but important, question of whether to add radiotherapy to chemotherapy when treating advanced Hodgkin's disease.

Treatment of Non-Hodgkin's Lymphomas

In contrast with Hodgkin's disease, non-Hodgkin's lymphomas are not always treated with the intention to cure. Certain patients fail to remain in complete remission despite treatment with surgery, radiation, or chemotherapy. We do not know why this happens. Perhaps the cells are resistant to treatment, or they may hide in sanctuary areas such as the brain or testes. The pathologist may predict from the biopsy which types of lymphoma are likely to behave this way, but the prediction is not anywhere near 100 percent certain.

Non-Hodgkin's lymphoma patients can be divided into two groups: those who may be cured by aggressive, although somewhat risky, chemotherapy with a combination of drugs; and those who are unlikely to be cured with the available drugs but can be treated over an extended period of time for relief of symptoms. With the currently available drugs, only certain subtypes of non-Hodgkin's lymphoma are likely to be cured, even with the best treatment. If you are diagnosed with non-Hodgkin's lymphoma, discuss with your oncologist and pathologist which subtype you have and what to expect with and without therapy.

One subtype is considered curable: more than 40 percent of patients with diffuse histiocytic lymphoma achieve complete remission for five years or more. On the other hand, a large number of patients are diagnosed with nodular non-Hodgkin's lymphomas. A laboratory examination of the diseased lymph node determines whether it has nodular characteristics. Under the microscope the malignant lymphocytes appear in distinct clusters called nodules. Patients with nodular tumors survive for many years with no treatment or with sequential treatment to relieve pain with one, two, or three drugs. Often, these patients remain free of symptoms, although their disease can be detected by physical examination or X rays. We are not yet sure why this subtype is considered incurable, since patients can remain free of symptoms with no treatment for many years. Unfortunately, they relapse before they are considered cured—five to ten years with no evidence of disease is considered a cure—and often their remission is only partial, that is, malignant cells can be found in their blood, bone marrow, or lymph nodes. Yet they have no symptoms.

If patients with nodular non-Hodgkin's lymphoma do have symptoms, they are minimal at first, but they can get progressively worse. In such cases, symptoms can be treated with drugs such as chlorambucil, cyclophosphamide, or prednisone, prescribed as a daily dose taken orally. Alternatively, a combination drug regimen (COP) consisting of intravenous or oral cyclophosphamide, intravenous Oncovin (vincristine), and prednisone successfully relieves symptoms of these slowly progressive malignancies. Side effects are usually minimal and may include moderate hair loss, tingling in fingers and toes, and some increased risk of bleeding and infection. Patients often respond quickly to relief of such symptoms as fever, weight loss, or night sweats. If, despite a favorable pathology examination and prognosis, the disease progresses rapidly, then single-agent therapy can and often is replaced with multiple-drug chemotherapy, similar to that used with diffuse histiocytic lymphoma. Still, this is an effort to minimize only the symptoms.

Many different drug combinations have been used to treat non-Hodgkin's lymphomas. All of the programs listed in Chapter 2 employ multiple drugs given in cycles and contain cyclophosphamide or a similar drug along with vincristine or vinblastine. Almost all employ adriamycin, because malignant lymphocytes, among other cells, are particularly susceptible to its lethal effects. Originally, C-MOPP was the program used to treat diffuse histiocytic lymphomas. But with the availability of adriamycin, CHOP (cyclophosphamide, adriamycin or hydroxydaunomycin, Oncovin, and prednisone) became standard therapy. There is some evidence that the more complex drug combinations are better than CHOP, provided that full doses are used and the administration schedule strictly followed.

Keep in mind that each of the programs listed in Chapter 2 has its own unique problems. For example, M-BACOP requires high doses of methotrexate, which, in turn, needs an antidote, leucovorin, to prevent severe side effects, like mouth ulcers or bone marrow failure (see Chapter 8).

With all of these chemotherapy treatments, uric acid may be deposited in the urinary tract and other metabolic abnormalities can occur, particularly if the tumor is highly sensitive to the action of the multiple drugs used. Uric acid is a waste product that accumulates when large numbers of cancer cells are killed. Since kidney failure can result, patients are pretreated with a drug called allopurinol (Xyloprim) to prevent this complication. This drug prevents uric acid from building up in the blood and should be used in all lymphoma patients before administration of combination chemotherapy. This drug can occasionally cause side effects, too—most often a skin rash and a low white cell count. A similar drug, oxypurinol (not FDA approved) is available from the manufacturer, Burroughs-Wellcome, for patients who are sensitive to allopurinol but require therapy to reduce uric acid accumulation.

Salvage therapy. Despite combination drug therapy, at least half the patients with diffuse histiocytic lymphoma ultimately relapse. In these cases, salvage therapy is used in a last-ditch attempt to treat the disease. Salvage therapy usually consists of treatment with one or more drugs, e.g., VP-16 or cisplatin, to which the patient has not been previously exposed. Almost always, such therapy is used only to relieve symptoms.

Autologous marrow transplantation. A more recent approach to salvage therapy and to treatment of lymphomas is autologous marrow transplantation (AMT). Patients who have relapsed are given large doses of drugs, such as cyclophosphamide, BCNU, or VP-16. The severe and potentially fatal side effects of these drugs on the bone marrow would normally prevent their use. However, prior to drug treatment, samples of the patient's own bone marrow are removed and stored frozen in liquid nitrogen. Then, after chemotherapy treatment, it is injected back into the patient. The cells re-enter the marrow, proliferate, and resume production of normal red cells, white cells, and platelets. Techniques are available to "clean up" the patient's marrow, removing lymphoma cells before injecting it back into the patient. This clean-up procedure is experimental and is currently performed only as part of strictly monitored clinical trials. Eventually, however, the procedure may be used to cure lymphomas with good prognosis. (See Chapter 8 for a full discussion of bone marrow transplantation.)

Acute and Chronic Leukemias

The diagnosis of leukemia is one of those most feared by the public, bringing up images of early death, associated with a great deal of pain and suffering. Actually, some forms of leukemia show no symptoms for years and are slow to kill. There are more than twenty different kinds of leukemia. All are malignancies involving the various types of white cells of the blood, cells that normally protect our bodies from infection and provide a number of other life-maintaining functions. White blood cells are produced in the bone marrow, where they mature and then are released into the blood. But when one kind of white cell becomes malignant, it multiplies at an uncontrolled rate in the bone marrow, immature cells are released into the blood and other organs, and the cells become ineffective in their protective role.

Except for one chronic type, leukemia is a rare disease, so that details concerning treatment with chemotherapy would be of interest to only a relative few. It should be stressed, however, that many of the advances in treating other types of cancer with drugs resulted from research into therapy for leukemia. It is hoped that many of the strides made in curing some forms of leukemia with chemotherapy will be repeated with other much more common diseases, such as lung and colon cancers.

There are four common types of leukemia: acute lymphocytic, acute myelocytic, chronic lymphocytic, and chronic myelocytic.

Acute Lymphocytic Leukemia (ALL)

Robert F., at the age of nine, developed multiple black-and-blue marks on his body. His pediatrician found his white blood cell count to be very high, with mostly young lymphocytes (sometimes referred to as "blast" cells) present. His platelet count was very low, accounting for the black-and-blue marks. He was diagnosed with common acute lymphocytic leukemia (cAll) when larger than normal numbers of blasts were found in his bone marrow specimen. Before starting chemotherapy, he was given allopurinol to protect his kidneys from being damaged by uric aid, a cell breakdown product. Weekly intravenous doses of vincristine and daunomycin were administered to avoid pain and tissue damage that can occur if the drug spills into the tissues surrounding the vein. He took daily doses of oral prednisone. His blood cell counts were carefully monitored over the next four weeks. When the malignant cells disappeared from his bloodstream, another bone marrow specimen was taken from his pelvic bone. It showed a normal number of blasts and other young lymphocytes. Doses of the drug methotrexate were injected into his spinal fluid and radiation was administered to his testicles. Maintenance therapy with methotrexate and 6-mercaptopurine was continued for thirty months. He remained in complete remission, with normal bone marrow examinations and normal blood counts.

Four years after the diagnosis was made, when he was thirteen, malignant cells were discovered in his blood, and his bone marrow again supported the diagnosis of leukemia. Complete remission was again obtained with a program similar to that used previously. This time, however, treatment was more intensive and included two new drugs, adriamycin and asparaginase. At this point, he underwent bone marrow transplantation using donor bone marrow from his brother. Before receiving the transplant, he was subjected to large doses of radiation and cyclophosphamide to destroy all remaining malignant cells. These doses would normally be fatal, but they destroy residual malignant cells, and the transplanted bone marrow ultimately restores normal blood counts. For six weeks he was in an intensive care isolation unit, receiving blood transfusions, antibiotics, and drugs to prevent his body from rejecting the transplanted marrow. He finally recovered and has remained free of leukemia for the past five years and probably is cured.

Lymphocytic leukemias are closely related to malignant lymphomas. Here, too, lymphocytes become malignant but, rather than accumulating in the lymph nodes, the blood and bone marrow fill up with cells, interfering with production of normal red and white cells. Malignant lymphomas of the lymph nodes and lymphocytic leukemias of the blood and marrow frequently overlap. Some patients, for example, will have lymphoma cells in their enlarged lymph nodes and also large numbers of the same or similar cells circulating in their blood.

ALL is the usual type of leukemia afflicting children up to fifteen years of age (about 2,000 new cases are diagnosed each year). These children often come to the attention of their doctors because of infections or bleeding. ALL is generally diagnosed by examining blood and bone marrow cells under a microscope. Although some patients have extremely low white blood cell counts, it is more common for them to have high white cell counts with higher than normal numbers of lymphocytes in their blood. Very young, early-stage lymphocytes, normally seen only in the bone marrow, also appear in the blood. These early cells, called lymphoblasts, may spread into important organs such as the liver and lymph nodes, interfering with the function of those organs.

Before modern therapy evolved, ALL was usually quickly fatal. Patients with ALL ultimately died from infection, bleeding, or failure of a major organ. Today, chemotherapy is universally accepted as the treatment of choice for children and also for adults who develop ALL. After the diagnosis is made, the patient's cells are studied by using several techniques. How they look under the microscope, the nature of the proteins (antigens) on the cell surfaces, and certain other properties enable oncologists to subtype ALL patients into several different categories. To some extent, the intensity of chemotherapy is determined by the subtype.

The most common subtype of ALL is called common ALL (cALL), the type with which Robert F. was diagnosed. As I described in Robert's case study, it is treated in a rather standard manner, but new variations are always being tried in attempts to increase the cure rate, which is now 80 percent. Also, more attention is being paid to giving salvage chemotherapy to patients who fail initial drug therapy and to developing more complex treatments, such as bone marrow transplants, for the less common and sometimes more difficult-to-cure ALL subtypes.

Chemotherapy for ALL is begun with one of two drug combinations: vincristine, daunomycin (or adriamycin), and prednisone; or vincristine, prednisone, and methotrexate. This initial therapy, lasting about one month, is called the induction phase. Vincristine is administered intravenously each week; the adrenal corticosteroid prednisone is taken orally each day; and the methotrexate is given either intravenously or orally at different intervals, depending on the specific treatment program. Blood is drawn frequently for cell counts, and a bone marrow aspiration may be done for examination when the patient seems to be in remission. A bone marrow aspiration is a relatively painless nonsurgical procedure for drawing a small specimen of marrow from the breastbone or the pelvic bone of the hip. Infants, however, may undergo a surgical procedure to take marrow from the spine. If complete remission is reached, blood counts return to normal or near normal, and the bone marrow again produces normal percentages of young cells. If remission is not likely to be reached with just these two or three drugs, then either adriamycin (or daunomycin), asparaginase, or both are added to the program. If a patient has a subtype with a poorer prognosis than cALL, these same drugs may be used as part of the initial induction therapy. Unfortunately, asparaginase may produce severe allergic reactions, fever, vomiting, or other abnormal bodily functions. Adriamycin or daunomycin is, therefore, preferred.

Once complete remission is obtained, treatment is directed at so-called sanctuary sites, where malignant cells can hide and be relatively safe from the effects of drug therapy. The testes in boys are common sites that must be further treated with radiation to obtain complete remission. Unfortunately, this treatment makes them sterile. The central nervous system, which consists of the brain and the spinal cord, is another sanctuary site. These sites are commonly treated by directing X rays at the entire brain and by infusing methotrexate or cytosine arabinoside into the spinal fluid. The drugs are given through a needle passed through the skin into the spinal column or by an Omaya reservoir implanted in the scalp with a catheter running into the fluid-containing space surrounding the brain. Unfortunately, in some children these treatments can cause some impairment of brain function, perhaps less so with drugs given into the spinal fluid than with radiation to the brain. Symptoms of damage include decreased performance on standardized testing and some loss of learning ability, memory, and physical coordination. Special education classes directed at the patient's learning disability can help improve performance, and physical therapy can help correct coordination problems.

The purpose of all this treatment is to drastically lower the number of malignant cells in the patient's body. It is believed that once this is done, the body's own defenses can destroy any remaining malignant cells. Although we are not sure of the mechanism, these chemotherapy treatments do render ALL patients free of disease. For a period of time, say, thirty months, these children receive maintenance chemotherapy with the same or different drugs, such as 6-mercaptopurine, cytosine arabinoside, teniposide, cyclophosphamide, or methotrexate at various doses. Methotrexate sometimes requires use of an antidote, leucovorin, to prevent severe side effects (see Chapter 8). Many types of salvage chemotherapy programs are available for patients who relapse or do not obtain full remission, but salvage programs are much less likely than initial therapy to result in relapse-free remission.

Although drugs are chosen so that their side effects do not over-lap, hair loss, infection, bleeding, mouth sores (inflammation of the gums, tongue, and mouth lining), gastrointestinal upset, and nerve pains are common. Except for the hair loss, these side effects may be minimal or even absent in many of the children treated with the less intensive programs. More unusual side effects may also occur (see Chapter 2).

Chemotherapy for ALL disrupts the bone marrow by suppress-ing normal blood cells as well as malignant ones. Side effects re-sulting from low blood cell counts can be severe. A bone marrow transplant may help patients who relapse or do not enter remission by restoring blood cell production. The marrow may be taken from a donor or, before chemotherapy begins, it can be taken from the patient for use later on (see Chapter 8).

Acute Myelocytic Leukemia

Mr. D., age sixty, felt weak and exhausted. His physician found him to be anemic. His platelet count was low and his white blood cell count was ten times normal, with many malignant granulocytes present. Because of the increased risk of bleeding into the brain or other organs, chemotherapy was started immediately after a bone marrow sample was obtained and analyzed. A large dose of hydroxyurea, a drug that rapidly reduces the number of malignant cells in the blood without significantly affecting normal cells in the bone marrow, was administered orally. This brought his white cell count down to only twice the normal level. He was then given standard continuous intravenous induction therapy with daunomycin for three days and cytosine arabinoside for seven days.

Over the next ten days, his white cell count fell to nearly zero, his platelets dropped to an equally dangerous level, and he required red cell and platelet transfusions every other day. On the tenth day after treatment was started, his temperature rose abruptly to 105 degrees and he went into shock. He was suffering from a blood infection requiring multiple antibiotics and surgical drainage of an abscess in his rectal area. He recovered from the infection, and a subsequent bone marrow examination showed about 10 percent residual malignant cells. A short course of chemotherapy with three days of cytosinc arabinoside and one day of daunomycin was complicated by severe painful mucositis (inflammation and ulceration of gums, tongue, and lining of the mouth). Herpes simplex virus was cultured from the mouth ulcers, and he was treated with acyclovir, an antiviral antibiotic, to relieve his symptoms.

One more course of drugs, identical to the second, was given without complication. After his blood counts and bone marrow had returned to normal, four cycles of intravenous maintenance therapy were given. One cycle of cytosine arabinoside and daunomycin was administered every three weeks on an outpatient basis. On two occasions, he required hospitalization for fevers and infections when his white blood cell count fell to less than one-fifth of normal. Currently, his blood counts are again normal, eighteen months since the original diagnosis of leukemia was made.

In contrast with acute lymphocytic leukemia (ALL), which primarily affects children, acute myelocytic leukemia (AML) primarily affects adults, though some young adults are diagnosed with the condition. The malignant cells in AML are very young forms of the granulocyte, a type of white blood cell that protects the body from bacteria and other infections. These young forms are called myeloblasts.

It is easy to diagnose AML by examining the blood and bone marrow. Unfortunately, we do not have drugs that will kill only the malignant granulocytes. The normal granulocytes, therefore, are also destroyed, causing severe side effects. But, with present-day chemotherapy, approximately 20 percent of adult patients with this type of leukemia can be cured—but not without risk. Almost all go through a phase of bone marrow aplasia, that is, the normal blood cells will not be produced, and the patient will become extremely vulnerable to infection and bleeding.

Standard therapy employs two drugs, cytosine arabinoside and daunomycin, both given intravenously. Cytosine arabinoside is continuously infused, and daunomycin is injected daily for three days. Then the cytosine arabinoside is continued for another four days. Because continuous infusion is required, the patient must be hospitalized. This procedure is called an induction course, that is, a program of chemotherapy designed to eliminate malignant cells from the patient's marrow. For the next ten days to two weeks, the patient's blood counts will fall to dangerous levels, requiring transfusions of red cells to correct anemia and platelets to prevent serious bleeding. In some treatment centers, antibiotics are given to prevent infection, but if fever or other signs of infection occur, antibiotics are almost always required.

Allopurinol is used, as in ALL, to prevent kidney damage from uric acid, a cell breakdown product. If all goes well, the number of malignant cells in the blood will decrease and normal cells will be restored. At this point, another bone marrow examination is performed. If it shows that the malignant cells are no longer present in significant numbers, then one more course of cytosine arabinoside and daunomycin is given, followed by several cycles of chemotherapy with drugs such as adriamycin, azacytidine, prednisone, 6-mercaptopurine, methotrexate, or vincristine. In some patients, several induction courses with cytosine arabinoside and daunomycin are required in order to obtain a complete remission. Approximately 80 percent of adult AML patients will go into complete remission with chemotherapy, but only a fraction can be maintained disease-free for a prolonged period of time.

Various modifications of this program are employed to treat the subtypes of AML, such as promyelocytic leukemia (which sometimes requires blood thinners at the time of induction to prevent abnormal clotting), monocytic leukemia (monocytes are also white blood cells, developing from the same early cells as granulocytes), and erythroleukemia (abnormalities of red cells as well as granulocytes).

In contrast with ALL, maintenance chemotherapy for AML is administered for only a few monthly cycles. Another advantage is that there is no need to take measures to prevent cells from spreading to the brain or spinal fluid, because myeloblasts are rarely found in the spinal fluid or brain of patients with AML. Because of the large number of infusions required for both ALL and AML, the patient is generally fitted early in the course of treatment with an indwelling catheter into a major vein. With an indwelling catheter, the vein is kept open and accessible for infusion or injection (see Chapter 8).

Bone marrow transplantation (BMT) is a relatively new and experimental option for the treatment of patients with AML (see Chapter 9). The way patients are selected for this procedure is currently undergoing change. At present, patients less than forty years old who have gone into complete remission with chemotherapy are suitable candidates to receive BMT. It is not yet clear whether patients who are older, or who are resistant to chemotherapy, will benefit from BMT. As transplant technology improves, bone marrow transplantation may eventually replace chemotherapy as primary treatment for AML.

Chronic Lymphocytic Leukemia

Chronic lymphocytic leukemia (CLL) is closely related to non-Hodgkin's lymphoma. In lymphoma, there is an excess number of lymphocytes in the patient's lymph nodes. In CLL, lymphocytes predominate in the blood and bone marrow. Of course, there are cases of lymphoma where malignant lymphocytes are present in the bloodstream as well as the lymph nodes. Conversely, patients with CLL may have lymph nodes that, under the microscope, are diagnosed as lymphoma.

Most patients with CLL are in their sixties or seventies. They usually have no symptoms at all, or they may have fevers, enlarged lymph nodes, bleeding, weight loss, or drenching night sweats. Often, patients find out they have CLL because their blood counts are abnormal when they go to the doctor for routine physical exams or for other medical problems. The disease is not yet curable, but it often progresses quite slowly, and the patients frequently die from other causes after living with the disease for years or even decades.

For patients who require therapy, many treatment programs exist. The choice of therapy depends on which type of CLL is present and on the patient's symptoms and ability to function. Chemotherapy programs range from the use of single agents given orally to complex regimens similar to those used to treat non-Hodgkin's lymphoma. It is important to recognize that all therapies currently available for CLL are intended to relieve symptoms and not intended to cure. Some patients may not need therapy for years. For each type of CLL, I will describe some of the more commonly used treatment programs.

Classical CLL is by far the most common form and is usually seen in older patients. Lymph nodes become enlarged, and an excess number of mature, normal-appearing lymphocytes appear in the blood. These lymphocytes are easily distinguished from the immature forms seen in acute lymphocytic leukemia. Because these patients often live for many years with the disease, treatment may be delayed until symptoms, such as fever, weight loss, or obstruction of vital organs, occur. Drugs such as chlorambucil or cyclophosphamide, given orally on a daily basis, will often shrink lymph nodes and relieve symptoms for years. There are few side effects, although some hair loss can be expected with cyclophosphamide. The bone marrow may be suppressed, requiring transfusions for anemia, antibiotics for infection, or treatment for bleeding, because of low platelet counts. In some cases, pretreatment with allopurinol is necessary to prevent uric acid crystals from forming in the urine, causing kidney failure. If the disease is more advanced or aggressive, vincristine or adrenal corticosteroids are added to alleviate symptoms. These more complex programs are similar to those used to treat non-Hodgkin's lymphoma.

Mr. O., at age eighty, noticed he was losing weight and went to see his internist. Examination revealed lymph node enlargement, and his white cell count was ten times normal. A consulting hematologist (leukemia specialist) found that 98 percent of his lymphocytes were of the mature type seen in CLL and made that diagnosis. Treatment was initiated with five tablets per day of chlorambucil and then reduced to one per day when his lymphocyte count fell to near normal. Over a period of three months, Mr. O.'s appetite and weight returned to normal, his lymph nodes decreased to normal size, and his blood counts normalized except for anemia, which was considered to be caused by the drug. Until the dose of chlorambucil was reduced, he required transfusion of red cells to prevent dizziness and shortness of breath on exertion, symptoms of the drug-induced anemia. He remained on one or two pills of chlorambucil daily for three years without any other serious complications. Then, without warning, his lymph nodes began to enlarge again. A biopsy revealed the presence of a highly malignant form of non-Hodgkin's lymphoma, and he was started on multiple-drug chemotherapy. Again he went into clinical remission for eighteen months, but subsequently his old symptoms returned, and despite trials of other chemotherapeutic agents, he passed away from overwhelming infection.

Another type of CLL is actually a leukemic form of non-Hodgkin's lymphoma. The disease starts in the lymph nodes, as a lymphoma, but rapidly spreads to the blood and bone marrow. There it acts like CLL. Examination of the patient's blood by a pathologist, however, will show that the lymphocytes have certain characteristics that suggest the correct diagnosis. Since the two conditions are so similar, patients with this form of leukemia are treated with the same chemotherapy programs as those with non-Hodgkin's lymphoma.

Two highly malignant forms of CLL—acute lymphosarcoma cell-leukemia and prolymphocytic leukemia—are rare and require multiagent chemotherapy to relieve symptoms.

The fifth and last subtype of CLL is hairy cell leukemia, signified by the presence of an abnormal type of lymphocyte in the blood. Hairy cell lymphocytes have fine protrusions, like hairs, coming from their cell walls. The disease is rarely diagnosed. An immunomodulator drug, interferon, is approved by the FDA for treatment of newly diagnosed cases. Immunomodulators are chemicals that are normally produced by lymphocytes to regulate the body's defense mechanisms. Interferon is produced to defend against viral infections. It is now possible to manufacture large quantities of this naturally occurring chemical through the use of genetic engineering and gene-splicing techniques.

Treatment of hairy cell leukemia is begun when the first symptoms, such as infections or bleeding, appear. Therapy then consists of interferon, self-administered by injection under the skin, three times per week. Side effects include fever, uneasiness, and fatigue. These side effects can be mild at the dose level used to treat hairy cell leukemia, and they become even less severe as treatment continues. A second drug, deoxycoformycin (Pentostatin), is also highly effective. Some patients seem to respond favorably to interferon, while others respond better to deoxycoformycin.

It is often necessary to remove the patient's spleen when treating this disease. For some unknown reason, patients who undergo spleen removal respond better to chemotherapy than those who do not. The only disadvantages of removing the spleen are the usual risks of any operation and slightly increased risk of developing an infection.

Chronic Myelocytic Leukemia

Patients with chronic myelocytic leukemia (CML) tend to be elderly, although young adults do occasionally develop the disease. Most patients learn they have CML when they have routine blood counts for another purpose. Symptoms include excessive fatigue, abdominal discomfort from an enlarged spleen, or infections or bleeding as with other leukemias. An elevated white blood cell count and other characteristic blood abnormalities are all that is needed to make the diagnosis.

Patients are generally diagnosed during the early or stable phase of the disease. This phase of CML is treated easily with oral drugs, such as busulfan, hydroxyurea, phenylalanine mustard, or chlorambucil. A daily dose of drug is taken orally, and the dose is adjusted according to the results of blood counts done every two to three weeks at first and then every four to five weeks or longer if counts are stable. All these drugs have similar side effects related to the degree of effect on the bone marrow, and each one has certain side effects or problems more or less unique to itself. For example, busulfan can cause fiber deposits, called fibrosis, or scarring in the bone marrow, which can suppress bone marrow function for months. It can also cause darkening of the skin. Hydroxyurea often requires frequent dosage adjustments to prevent bone marrow suppression. Because leukemia rarely occurs following long-term use of hydroxyurea, this drug has recently been favored by many hematologists.

Despite the ease with which CML can be treated in its early stages, once it has transformed to its acute form the prognosis becomes very poor. After a stable period of three to five years a transformation occurs, resulting in a disease that closely resembles either acute myelocytic or acute lymphocytic leukemia. Once this happens, the patient is treated with therapy for the acute leukemia. Few patients achieve long-term remissions, and the most that can be expected is relief of symptoms. Most patients die within one year of this transformation.

Bone marrow transplants for early CML. Until recently, early CML could be treated only with chemotherapy. Today, however, bone marrow transplantation (BMT) has proven effective in preventing stable CML from transforming into acute leukemia, something that chemotherapy by itself could not. The downside is that some patients do not survive the complications of BMT (see Chapter 8).

It is difficult for a doctor to recommend BMT, with its risks, to a patient who at the time has few symptoms but will ultimately transform and die. Only by consulting with your oncologist can you determine what is right for you. At best, 50 to 80 percent of patients who undergo BMT will have long-term survival free of disease. The rest will die as a result of the BMT or relapse after BMT has been initially successful. Relapsed patients are difficult to treat because they have already received a great deal of chemotherapy, and most die of their disease, its complications, or from the complications of further chemotherapy.

Chemotherapy for advanced CML. In advanced CML, bone marrow transplantation is not very successful and is being done less and less. Patients who have transformed into ALL generally receive intravenous vincristine and oral prednisone, and sometimes intravenous adriamycin. About 70 percent of these patients will enter remission, with an average survival of one year. Patients who have transformed into AML receive intravenous daunomycin and cytosine arabinoside, but as a rule, these patients do even less well on chemotherapy than those with ALL transformation.

Testicular Cancer

Combination chemotherapy for cancer of the male testes cures 70 percent or more of patients with this rare tumor. Although several types of tumors can affect the testes, the prognosis is excellent for all of them. Patients initially go to the doctor because they have lumps in the testicles, or pain due to spread of the cancer to the liver or other organs.

The first step in treating these cancers is to surgically remove the tumor in the testes and nearby lymph nodes, if there is no distant spread at the time of diagnosis. One type of testicular cancer, called seminoma, is generally treated successfully with surgery and radiation. The other types, the most common one called embryonal, often require chemotherapy in addition to surgery and radiation.

The embryonal type of testicular tumor may secrete lactate dehydrogenase or alpha fetoprotein, substances released into the blood that can be used as markers to guide chemotherapy. Similarly, another type secretes human choriogonadotropin (HCG), which can be measured in the blood to monitor the progress of therapy. If these substances do not return to normal blood levels following chemotherapy treatment or if they again start to increase, further chemotherapy is usually needed. Patients with extensive disease have at least a 70 percent chance of cure with chemotherapy. Patients with less extensive disease can expect a cure rate of greater than 95 percent. There is, therefore, no reason for patients to refuse chemotherapy for treatment of testicular cancer.

If the disease has spread beyond the testes and lymph nodes or if surgery and radiation have not cured the seminoma type of testicular cancer, then combination chemotherapy must be employed. The treatment of choice is a combination of cisplatin, VP-16, and bleomycin (PVB) given in twenty-one-day cycles for a total of four cycles. Following chemotherapy, additional radiation or surgery may be required to destroy or remove residual disease. There are many variations of this program, employing different doses, schedules, and maintenance therapy.

Drug combinations other than PVB may also be used for initial treatment of testicular cancer. These include VAB VI (vinblastine, actinomycin, bleomycin, cyclophosphamide, and cisplatin) and PEB (cisplatin, etoposide, and bleomycin). To obtain the highest cure rates, it is necessary to administer full doses of the drugs in the PVB, PEB, or VAB VI programs, regardless of the low white blood cell and platelet counts that may result. Lower doses reduce the chances of curing the disease (see Chapter 7).

Patients who do not respond fully to initial therapy are given actinomycin, adriamycin, and etoposide to relieve symptoms and, occasionally, to provide long-term, disease-free survival. Ifosfamide, a drug related to cyclophosphamide, has recently been used, usually in combination with other drugs, to treat testicular cancers. It is given along with mesna, a drug that prevents ifosfamide from affecting the bladder and causing bleeding and painful urination. Studies are under way to determine which patients require more aggressive chemotherapy and which should receive smaller, less frequent doses.

Almost all patients with testicular cancer that has spread beyond the testes will become infertile as a result of the chemotherapy, radiation, and surgery needed to cure the disease. Nothing can be done to prevent this. Sperm banking can be done if patients wish to have children later on. Sperm is frozen prior to cancer treatment and defrosted later for insemination. Your oncologist can tell you how to locate commercial sperm banks. Unfortunately, however, few women become pregnant using this procedure, probably because, for some reason, patients with testicular cancer often have low sperm counts or poor sperm quality.

The following case illustrates the excellent results that can be obtained with combination chemotherapy of testicular cancer:

Mr. P. was found to have a mass in his right testicle. A biopsy proved it to be an embryonal carcinoma. Surgical exploration of his abdomen revealed that the tumor had spread to lymph nodes in his pelvis and abdomen. A metastatic tumor mass was also found near his kidney. Both tumor masses were surgically removed, but some tumor was obviously left behind. Following surgery, he was started on PVB combination chemotherapy. His alpha fetoprotein level fell from ten times normal to normal and no disease could be found on X-ray scanning. His complications included hair loss, nausea, and one serious infection, bacterial pneumonia, during a period when his white blood cell count fell to almost zero. Now, ten years after treatment, there has been no recurrence and, except for infertility, he is living a normal life.

Cancer of the Fetal Placenta (Choriocarcinoma)

The placenta is a spongy structure that forms in a woman's uterus during pregnancy as the means for nourishing the developing fetus. Although rare, a tumor arising from the placenta is highly curable. These malignant tumors are called choriocarcinomas. If the cancer has spread from the placenta into the surrounding uterus, that organ must be surgically removed. However, in many cases, combination chemotherapy can cure the disease without removing the uterus.

About 95 percent of choriocarcinomas that have not spread, or have spread only to the lungs, are curable with chemotherapy. Results are not as favorable if the tumor spreads to organs other than the lungs. We do not know why this is so.

Mrs. T. was thirty-eight years old and had two children. She became pregnant, but ultrasound examination showed that the fetus was abnormal. A D&C was done to scrape out the contents of her uterus. A pathological examination revealed the presence of choriocarcinoma, and a subsequent chest X ray showed that it had spread to the lungs. Assays of the hormone HCG in her blood (see below) were markedly elevated, far above levels seen with a normal pregnancy. After surgical removal of her uterus, she was started on combination chemotherapy with three drugs. Her HCG level dropped gradually until it became entirely normal. She received three more cycles of chemotherapy and, on follow-up over the next five years, had no recurrence of the cancer. Her chest X ray rapidly became normal and has remained so, as has her HCG level.

Choriocarcinomas produce a substance called human chorionic gonadotropin (HCG), a fact that helps achieve high cure rates. HCG is a hormone normally produced by the placenta in pregnant women, and its presence is the basis for pregnancy tests. If HCG is present at very high levels, it suggests the presence of choriocarcinoma, particularly if ultrasound examination of the uterus shows that the fetus is abnormal. Levels of HCG in the patient's blood are used to guide chemotherapy. That is, if the HCG level returns to normal and stays at normal levels for one to three months, treatment is stopped. If, despite treatment, the HCG level increases, the oncologist will reevaluate chemotherapy and perhaps change to another dosage or another drug.

Many factors are important to the oncologist in determining how chemotherapy should be used in individual patients. Because these tumors are rare, however, I describe one typical program that is often used to treat them if they are confined to the uterus or even if they have spread to the lungs or elsewhere.

The most commonly used program employs intravenous actinomycin for five days with repeat doses every two to three weeks; intravenous methotrexate for five days with repeat doses every two weeks; and oral chlorambucil. Treatment is continued until HCG levels return to normal, and then one to three more cycles of combination chemotherapy are administered. In advanced cases, where the tumor has spread to the brain or liver, or when disease has recurred after treatment, combination chemotherapy may be supplemented with radiation to the brain or other tumor sites. Long-term survival may be obtained by surgical removal of persistent tumors along with salvage chemotherapy. Ultimately, patients with advanced or recurrent choriocarcinoma have at least a 60 percent chance of a cure.

CHAPTER 6

Chemotherapy
to Help Quality of Life

Many common cancers cannot be cured by chemotherapy. When cure is impossible, patients may be given palliative chemotherapy, intended to lessen the pain or make the disease less severe. It is given in the hope of improving the quality of life and giving the patient the ability to carry on daily activities free of pain or discomfort.

Advanced Breast Cancer

Compared with hormone therapy, as described in Chapter 5, chemotherapy has more complications and often produces fewer long-lasting remissions. Therefore, hormone therapy is preferred as initial treatment for advanced breast cancer, unless the patient has large metastases in the liver and lungs, metastases in the brain, or no estrogen receptors on her tumor cells. Although chemotherapy for advanced breast cancer only relieves symptoms and does not cure the metastatic disease, it can make life less uncom-

111

fortable for many women who might otherwise be incapacitated. Thus, there is little reason not to recommend palliative chemotherapy for them.

Patients with advanced breast cancer receive drug treatments similar to those used as additive chemotherapy in early stages of the disease (see Chapter 5). The goal is to keep the patient comfortable and relieve symptoms caused by the tumor. Physicians usually wait for symptoms to develop before initiating drug therapy. These symptoms might be pain caused by spread of the tumor into the bones or liver, or difficulty breathing because of spread to the lungs. With some patients, however, it is clear that the cancer will progress, making it advisable to start therapy before obvious symptoms appear. For breast cancer patients, relieving pain, improving organ function, and preventing weight loss are among the important goals of palliative chemotherapy. There are too many palliation treatment programs for advanced breast cancer to describe them all, so I'll detail one reasonable program.

Those patients requiring palliative chemotherapy have usually already undergone initial treatment with surgery and/or radiation therapy. Often hormone therapy has been tried, too, for palliation, but it has either failed or is no longer effective. About 60 percent of advanced breast cancer patients can find relief with chemotherapy, but there is no consistently reliable test to predict who will and who will not respond. An estrogen receptor analysis of the cancer cells can help predict responsiveness to hormone therapy, but it does not help determine the patient's likely response to chemotherapy.

Mrs. S. developed a breast lump that proved to be malignant and, unfortunately, had spread to her liver. She complained of pain over her liver and weight loss. Her tumor was negative for estrogen receptors. Because of this finding and the presence of large tumor deposits in the liver, chemotherapy, rather than hormone therapy, was administered. She received doses of 5-fluorouracil and methotrexate intravenously on days one and eight of each monthly drug cycle, followed by fourteen days of oral cyclophosphamide. This cycle was repeated every four weeks for nineteen months. Symptoms were relieved and she gained fifteen pounds. Her only complications were hair loss, which regrew after nine months of therapy, and one bout of pneumonia, which responded quickly to antibiotics. Finally she developed painful metastases in her bones, and adriamycin therapy was substituted for CMF (cyclophosphamide, methotrexate, and 5-fluorouracil). It was decided to give the adriamycin weekly, in small intravenous doses, as this was less likely to cause heart complications than administering much higher doses every three weeks. She went on to have a pain-free remission for six months but then relapsed. Complications included severe hair loss and painful mouth ulcers. Following her relapse, heralded by bone pain and skin metastases, an internal catheter and reservoir was placed under the skin of her right chest. An external portable pump connected to the catheter was filled every two days with vinblastine, thereby giving a continuous infusion of this drug for five days every three weeks. For another six months, her disease was stable and she was able to function. Only one complication occurred, an infection at the tip of the catheter, which had been placed in the right atrium, or receiving chamber, of her heart. To cure the infection, the catheter was removed, and she was treated with antibiotics. After the infection subsided, a similar catheter was installed. When she relapsed for the fourth time with large, painful liver metastases, she chose to terminate chemotherapy treatments and substitute narcotics to control pain. She died shortly thereafter.

Most oncologists start palliative breast cancer chemotherapy with some version of the five-drug program described by Dr. Richard Cooper in the 1970s. This program uses five drugs given in three- or four-week cycles. These drugs were cyclophosphamide, methotrexate, 5-fluorouracil, vincristine, and prednisone. This program was the first apparently successful treatment for advanced breast cancer. Patients with bone pain, skin lesions, and even liver involvement improved and maintained their improvement over a period of months and even years. Today, similar results are obtained with only the three-drug CMF program (cyclophosphamide, methotrexate, and 5-fluorouracil). Various versions of this program have now become standard first-line chemotherapy for palliation of advanced breast cancer. Many schedules with differing drug dosages, cycle intervals, and routes of administration (e.g., oral or intravenous) have been tried, but they are all equally successful. Some oncologists have advocated the use of tamoxifen—the hormone treatment described in Chapter 5—and chemotherapy together to treat breast cancer. Recent evidence shows, however, that this combination is probably no more beneficial than hormone or chemotherapy alone.

A typical CMF program consists of relatively small doses of methotrexate and moderate doses of 5-fluorouracil given intravenously every four weeks, along with tablets of cyclophosphamide taken orally every day for two weeks. The therapy continues until the patient either relapses or develops side effects that prevent further administration. Typical side effects include hair loss; increased frequency of urination or blood in the urine from bladder irritation; infections due to a decline in the white blood cell count; and bleeding due to a decline in the blood platelet count. Obviously toxic effects attributable to the individual drugs in the treatment program can occur (see Chapter 2).

Many oncologists have modified the CMF program, dropped the methotrexate, and added the drug adriamycin to it (CAF). Both programs are equally effective for symptom relief, but adriamycin is sometimes saved for use as a single drug when the tumor becomes resistant to CMF. Although adriamycin can also lower white cell and platelet counts, its main toxic effect is on the heart. After the patient receives more than seven hundred milligrams of the drug, heart failure may result. Heart failure occurs when the pumping action of the heart no longer works properly, in this case because the drug has a toxic effect on heart muscle. Symptoms of heart failure include shortness of breath, accumulation of fluid in the lungs and legs, and irregular heartbeats. Heart complications can be successfully treated, but the drug must be discontinued. This side effect is well known, and oncologists continually monitor patients with physical exams and special scans looking for any signs of heart failure. Recently, risk of this complication has been reduced by giving smaller doses of adriamycin on a weekly basis rather than large doses every three weeks.

Many patients are kept comfortable and functioning despite their cancer and the side effects of their drug therapy. Sooner or later, however, they relapse. Their quality of life deteriorates, and they are less able to carry on activities of daily living, such as keeping themselves clean, shopping and cooking, going out with friends, or taking care of financial responsibilities. This progresses to the point where they become bedridden and all their needs must be supplied by others. At this point, patients receive more complicated and usually more toxic chemotherapy.

One program employs the drug vinblastine. For best results, continuous infusion of this chemical into the bloodstream may be necessary. Steps are taken to prevent this very irritating drug from leaking into the skin at the site where the needle enters the vein. A permanent catheter is placed through an opening in the chest and tunneled into the patient's vein. To infuse the drug, a needle is inserted into a reservoir implanted under the skin and connected to the catheter.

Inserting the catheter is relatively simple and painless. However, it is necessary to maintain the catheter and to prevent it from becoming a site for serious infections. With the catheter in place, the patient can tolerate having the drug infused continuously for five days. In the past, patients had to be admitted to the hospital to receive this drug by special pumps hooked into their catheters. Now, however, smaller portable pumps, carried inconspicuously under the clothing, slowly infuse vinblastine into the indwelling catheter. Attempts are currently under way to develop a portable pump that will use greatly diluted drug, eliminating the need for an internal catheter.

If a patient relapses following vinblastine therapy, remission is not likely. At this point, the patient and family must decide whether to continue with less-tolerated and less-effective drugs (e.g., mitomycin, mitoxantrone, or high-dose methotrexate) or to proceed to experimental therapies, such as autologous marrow transplantation (AMT). If chemotherapy is chosen, the patient might respond with improved quality of life, at least for a short time. More likely, however, she will get side effects, depending on the drug used, and no useful benefit. In fact, her life might be shortened. If AMT is chosen, the same problem exists. The procedure is experimental and has lots of side effects (see Chapter 8), but there is some chance for a long-term remission.

One experimental approach to treating patients with far advanced breast cancer is the use of AMT plus chemotherapy consisting of some of the following drugs: BCNU, cyclophosphamide, VP-16, thiotepa, cisplatin, or carboplatin. Normally, intensive use of these drugs is not possible because they severely affect the patient's bone marrow, interfering with the production of blood cells. However, by obtaining marrow from the patient before beginning intensive chemotherapy, freezing it in liquid nitrogen to store it, and infusing it back intravenously into the patient, these usually fatal side effects of intensive chemotherapy can be avoided. The normal marrow restores blood production that was destroyed by the chemotherapy. (See Chapter 8 for a full description of the AMT procedure.) For breast cancer patients, it does not appear necessary to "clean up" the patient's marrow before returning it to the patient. That is, it is not necessary to use some technique to destroy any breast cancer cells that might be present in the marrow. Patients with obvious bone marrow metastases, however, may not be able to be treated by this experimental procedure because of the high risk of infusing tumor cells back into the patient with the reinfused marrow.

To date, results with AMT are encouraging, but long-term survival rates and the expected length of remissions are unknown, since this is a relatively new procedure. Keep in mind that by no means has this technique replaced standard chemotherapy. Patients suffer greatly during the aplastic phase and some die. For the time being, autologous marrow transplantation with extremely high doses of chemotherapy can be recommended only when all else has failed—or is likely to do so—or as part of a clinical trial.

Colon Cancer

Located at the lower end of the digestive tract, the colon, or large bowel, converts liquid wastes into solid fecal matter. The colon is a muscular tubelike structure that begins in the right lower side of the abdomen, rises to the ribs, continues across the abdomen, descends along the left side into the pelvis, and terminates at the anus. The portion of the colon located in the pelvis just before the anus is known as the rectum. Cancer cells grow silently in the lining of the colon and spread through the wall into nearby lymph glands and then into the liver, lungs, or brain. In fact, many tumors that appear to be liver cancer are actually colon cancers that have spread to the liver. The colon's large size, location near other organs, and its ability to distend or stretch allow cancer cells to grow and spread easily without being detected, contributing to the high death rate from colon cancer.

Screening and Diagnosis

Colon cancer generally appears in patients over fifty, but even young adults can develop it. It occurs equally in men and women. A screening test can be done using stool samples to look for blood loss. Procedures for passing tubes into the lower colon (sigmoidoscopy) or the whole colon (colonoscopy) can also be done to look for and remove growths or polyps, which over a period of years may become cancerous. It is not clear how often these procedures should be done. If you have no family history of colon cancer, a yearly screen of stool samples for blood is probably sufficient. Samples can be obtained at home and mailed to your physician for testing, or your physician may give you a test kit to use at home. Alternatively, your physician can do a sigmoidoscopy every three to five years. If you have a close relative with colon cancer, you should be tested more often and more thoroughly. In any case, whether you have a family history of colon cancer or not, you should see your doctor for X rays, colonoscopy, or sigmoidoscopy if you have any rectal bleeding or change in bowel habits.

Treatment

Complete surgical removal remains the only hope for curing colon cancer. At the time of operation, the surgeon removes the cancerous growth along with normal surrounding tissue. If the cancer is confined to the lining of the colon, the operation is almost 100 percent successful. Once the tumor spreads beyond what can be safely removed by operation, the patient's prognosis becomes very poor. If the wall of the large bowel is involved, the cure rate falls to seven out of ten, or only three out of ten if the tumor has spread into nearby lymph glands. The location of this tumor and resistance to treatment are primary reasons why it is the second most common fatal cancer.

Mrs. O. is sixty-nine years old. She discovered blood in her bowel movements, and X rays showed a rectal cancer. The surgeon removed the tumor, which was about to cause obstruction. He discovered signs of tumor throughout her abdomen and liver. Three months after surgery she reported pain and swelling in her abdomen. She and her family decided to accept chemotherapy rather than the alternative, narcotics. She received an injection of 5-fluorouracil (5FU) daily for five days every five weeks and obtained complete relief of pain two months after treatment ended. Nausea and occasional vomiting occurred after her treatments. Now, one year after starting 5FU therapy, she remains pain-free, although tests show the continued presence of tumor in her liver and abdomen. Perhaps 20 percent of patients with some malignancies can expect to live more than one year. Therefore, Mrs. O. will probably live no more than another year.

Even patients with incurable disease have the colon tumor removed to prevent obstruction of the digestive tract and uncontrollable vomiting. Currently available chemotherapy cannot destroy the remaining cancer cells, preventing a total cure if surgery is unsuccessful. For this reason, chemotherapy may relieve pain and suffering, but it cannot cure the disease.

Cancer pain is often caused by tumors pressing on nerves or on sensitive organs such as bones, or by the infiltration of the tumor into organs, expanding their sensitive capsules or coverings. For example, infiltration of a tumor into the liver causes tension on the thin capsule lining the liver. The capsule is sensitive to stretch, thereby resulting in pain. Similarly, obstruction caused by tumors of the bowel or the bile ducts, which drain the liver, results in pain. Here, the smooth muscle of the bowel or bile ducts contracts against the obstruction, resulting in severe cramping pain. Presumably chemotherapy slows the growth of tumor cells, relieving or postponing signs and symptoms due to this pressure or infiltration.

Only one drug, 5-fluorouracil (5FU), destroys enough colon cancer cells to lessen the pain experienced by patients with advanced colon cancer. After its introduction in the early 1960s, great enthusiasm developed for using 5FU in patients whose disease had spread beyond what surgery could safely remove. Physicians administered thousands of doses in response to reports that shrinkage of tumors occurred in up to 80 percent of patients with advanced colon cancer. We now know that less than two in ten patients actually benefit from this drug. The benefits include: (1) delay in the onset of pain caused when the tumor obstructs or infiltrates into other organs; (2) slowing of infiltration into organs such as the liver so that normal functioning is not affected; and (3) relief of obstruction of bile ducts so that bile can drain, relieving the patient's jaundice, or yellow skin color. Jaundice also causes severe itching as bile backs up into the skin. Treatment may prevent the jaundice or itching, at least for a while. However no one is cured, and benefits usually last only a few months. Despite this pessimistic outlook, 5FU continues to be used because no substitute exists and because patients tolerate its side effects. Other more or less dangerous drugs, such as nitrosoureas, leucovorin, cisplatin, and mitomycin (listed in Chapter 2), have been administered with 5FU, but long-term results are no better than with 5FU alone.

Drug companies supply 5FU in a solution that is administered over a five- to ten-minute period into a vein. Leakage into tissues around the site of injection may cause pain, redness, or swelling. Patients usually receive intravenous injections of the drug for five days every five or six weeks.

Physicians monitor both toxic and beneficial effects of 5FU by recording the patient's reports of side effects, by following up with regular physical examinations, and by performing laboratory blood tests. Patients may experience nausea, vomiting, diarrhea, or painful mouth ulcers. The physician may detect changes in the tumor masses during a physical examination. If the white blood cell count falls, the physician will decrease the drug dose and administer it less frequently. There is also a blood test for CEA, carcinoembryonic antigen, a protein substance which, if found in the blood of an adult, is thought to indicate the continued presence of colon cancer. CEA increases or decreases in concentration as colon cancer progresses or regresses. Rising values indicate further spread; falling values show a beneficial effect of chemotherapy.

Investigators have not yet discovered any new drugs that have promise against colon cancer. Only a major breakthrough will improve the prognosis of these patients. One experimental drug, FUDR (5-fluorodeoxyuridine), which is chemically related to 5FU, treats painful colon cancer that has spread primarily to the liver. A pump, sometimes implanted beneath the patient's skin, delivers the drug directly to the blood supply of the liver. No patients are cured, but one in three patients receives some relief from pain. Recently similar pumps, worn externally, have been used to deliver 5FU continuously through a catheter into a vein in the arm or chest. This catheter delivers the drug to the whole circulation, not just to the blood supply of the liver, but has the advantage of not requiring surgical implantation. Some investigators report better results by delivering 5FU with a catheter method than with standard intravenous injections every five or six weeks. Potential side effects are greater, however, since the catheter is a foreign body, and, therefore, a possible site of infection. The case history of Dr. R. illustrates the use of these new procedures.

Dr. R. developed a lump below his right ribs. X rays revealed a tumor in the colon, and surgical exploration showed a large mass in his liver. After removal of the colon cancer, the liver tumor grew and caused severe pain. Dr. R. elected to have a catheter threaded through his arteries into the blood supply of the liver. A small portable pump delivered a drug called 5-fluorodeoxyuridine (FUDR) into the catheter, enabling him to survive pain-free for one year. No serious side effects occurred. He later relapsed, and attempts to palliate with another drug failed. Progression of the liver tumor caused his death.

No adequate chemotherapy exists today for colon cancer that has spread beyond surgical care. Pain can be relieved with morphine sulfate either as a tablet taken orally or as an intravenous medication. Antiemetics such as thorazine or compazine can be used to relieve nausea or vomiting. They can be given orally, intravenously, or as a rectal suppository. Except for drowsiness, there are few serious side effects. These drugs relieve symptoms but do not affect the overall dismal prognosis. Patients with advanced disease face a very difficult choice. They can choose to relieve symptoms such as pain and vomiting with painkillers and antiemetics or they can undergo therapy with 5FU, which has unpleasant side effects, is expensive, and rarely brings long-term benefit. Pain relief with 5FU results from shrinkage of the tumor, not from a direct effect on pain. Despite the risks and costs of using this drug, about 20 percent of patients receiving 5FU will experience pain relief or relief from an obstructed bowel.

Very recently, reports have emerged concerning the use of 5FU and the drug levamisole (previously used to treat diseases caused by parasites) in patients with certain colon cancers, particularly those that had not spread through the bowel wall but were more advanced than just involving the colon lining. A statistically significant improvement in long-term survival (15 or 20 percentage points) was reported in patients treated with 5FU and levamisole soon after surgical removal of the tumor, compared to patients who had only surgical removal of the malignancy. This additive use of chemotherapy seems reasonable, but further studies are needed to confirm that this combination of drugs is truly beneficial. In addition, some oncologists have been recommending 5FU therapy with or without levamisole as additive therapy for all stages of colon cancers, especially those in the lower part of the colon. It is unlikely that these 5FU combinations will dramatically prevent colon cancer from spreading, since 5FU is not very active against colon tumors.

Lung Cancer

The lungs are two cone-shaped organs contained in the chest cavity. They are responsible for the function of respiration, by which the body takes in oxygen and releases carbon dioxide waste. Lung cancer is one of the more common malignancies and, unfortunately, its cure rate is only about 10 percent or less. For tumors confined to the lung, surgery and radiation hold some hope of cure. All too often, however, the disease has spread to distant sites and is not treatable by these methods. At this point, any chemotherapy is usually intended to relieve symptoms and not to cure.

The chemotherapy used to treat this disease depends on the type of lung cancer. There are three major types of lung cancer, each of which is named for the type of cell involved in the malignancy. These types are: squamous cell, adenocarcinoma, and small cell carcinoma. The diagnosis is made based on microscopic examination of the tumor itself or of cells shed by the tumor that are coughed up or obtained by a procedure called bronchoscopy. During bronchoscopy, a long tube is inserted into the throat and guided into the airways of the lung, where fluid secretions can be sampled or a brush can be used to obtain tumor cells.

Squamous Cell Cancer

This is the most common type of lung cancer. The cancer cells resemble squamous cells, the flat, scaly cells covering the skin and organ surfaces. If the tumor is confined to one lung and has not spread to adjacent lymph nodes or other structures, such as the space between the lungs or the outer lining of the lung, then surgery sometimes combined with radiation may cure the disease. Unhappily, however, once this type of cancer has spread beyond one lung, the chance for a long-term remission is very small.

Initial attempts to treat squamous cell cancer with chemotherapy were not successful. Today, however, there are several experimental programs involving combinations of two or more of the following drugs: cyclophosphamide, adriamycin, cisplatin, 5-fluorouracil, methotrexate, VP-16, vincristine, vindesine, and bleomycin. Still, it remains to be seen whether these experimental drug programs will affect the dismal cure rates or, at least, improve quality of life for patients with this disease.

Adenocarcinoma

Adenocarcinoma is a malignancy of cells that secrete substances. These cells are found in many different organs. In the lung, they line the bronchial tubes leading into the air sacs, where oxygen passes into the bloodstream. This type of lung cancer also benefits little from chemotherapy. Drugs like those used for squamous cell lung cancer yield few responses that last longer than a few weeks or months. FAM therapy (5-fluorouracil, adriamycin, and mitomycin) currently heads the list of available treatment, but long-term results are not good. Many other schedules and programs are being tried, including administration of CAP (cisplatin, adriamycin, and cyclophosphamide). However, until more effective drugs are found, there is little hope that the cure rate or chances of survival will improve.

Adenocarcinomas starting in other organs can mimic lung cancer. For example, cancers from the thyroid, breast, kidney, pancreas, or colon can spread to the lung and look like lung cancer, even under the microscope. Before beginning any chemotherapy for adenocarcinoma of the lung, therefore, it is crucial to determine if any other primary cancer is present. A primary cancer is the original tumor site, from which secondary, or metastatic, tumors arise. On occasion, a more effective hormonal or drug therapy exists for a metastatic tumor than for a primary lung cancer. For example, a lung tumor that has spread from an adenocarcinoma of the breast could be treated with a good chance of remission and few side effects; a similar tumor, originating in the lung, however, is much more difficult to treat. The presence of adenocarcinoma in other parts of the body can be determined in several ways. A tumor of the breast can be detected by breast examination and by mammography, an X-ray examination of the breast. A test for blood in the stool (feces) can sometimes indicate the presence of cancer in the colon. Physical examination of the ovary or prostate gland as well as the thyroid glands may be used to screen for most other adenocarcinomas.

Small Cell (Oat Cell) Carcinoma

Small cell carcinoma differs from other lung cancers in that it behaves more like a lymphoma (cancer of the lymph nodes) or leukemia (cancer of the white blood cells) than a malignancy of the lung. Like lymphoma and leukemia, small cell carcinoma responds to treatment. The disease often affects the bone marrow, like lymphoma and leukemia. When treated with chemotherapy or radiation, the disease will often completely regress for a period of months or even a year or two, only to reappear later as a fatal illness. It is unclear where small cells originate, but, when viewed under the microscope, they are definitely different in appearance from squamous or adenocarcinoma cells. This type of lung cancer may be diagnosed by examining a sample of lung tissue (biopsy) or, more often, by examining cells coughed up or obtained during bronchoscopy.

Many drugs and combinations of drugs, with radiotherapy, will totally destroy small cell carcinoma for a period of months or even years. A small percentage of patients are actually cured or at least have five- or ten-year remissions. Initial treatment is usually radiotherapy. A tumor confined to one lung and nearby lymph nodes is called limited stage disease. For this condition, chemotherapy combined with radiation is preferred, because controlled studies have shown that about 20 percent of patients treated with both chemotherapy and radiation at this stage survive longer or may even be cured. Sometimes, surgeons need only to remove a small primary tumor to cure the patient. Many oncologists believe, however, that surgery for other than the most limited disease should be avoided. If the disease has spread to areas outside the affected lung or returns after initial treatment, chemotherapy can be used to relieve symptoms.

Generally, limited stage small cell cancer of the lung is treated with radiotherapy and chemotherapy in an effort to cure the disease. The largest potential problem is that this tumor tends to spread silently to other organs, such as the brain and bone marrow. Metastasis to the brain is especially troublesome, since the brain is relatively immune to the effects of chemotherapy administered by mouth or by vein. Tumor cells may therefore hide in the brain tissue and grow even after apparently successful treatment. If the disease spreads to the bone marrow, it is then considered extensive, rather than limited, and there is virtually no hope of a cure with chemotherapy. In these cases, patients are given palliative chemotherapy to relieve symptoms.

Because of these problems when disease spreads to the brain or bone marrow, certain tests are routinely done before aggressive chemotherapy is even considered. To determine if the cancer is or is not a limited disease, a bone marrow sample (biopsy) and computer-assisted tomography (CAT) scan of the brain are typically performed. Furthermore, many oncologists use radiation to the brain as a preventive measure during or after lung cancer treatment. It is uncertain whether brain radiotherapy improves the cure rate, and the procedure does have side effects. For example, vomiting and hair loss may result, and rarely patients may suffer memory loss or impaired reasoning over the long run.

Practically every cancer drug is effective against small cell carcinoma of the lung, and there are so many different combinations and schedules in use that it is almost impossible to list them all. Usually, however, treatment involves two to four drugs, for example, cyclophosphamide, adriamycin, and cisplatin. Methotrexate, procarbazine, 5-fluorouracil, mitomycin C, vindesine, and vincristine are other common possibilities. Treatment generally lasts three to six months, and maintenance therapy does not seem to improve survival. Maintenance therapy, in this case, is chemotherapy given to keep a patient in complete remission after successful initial treatment. Often drugs can cause all detectable disease to disappear, but no drugs can prevent relapse. This is particularly true with small cell carcinoma of the lung. Many drugs can be used to obtain a remission, but most patients (80 percent or more) relapse in one year no matter what maintenance therapy is used.

Side effects depend on the drugs used and how doses are scheduled, but most are easily tolerated. More intense treatments will cause more severe side effects. Severe infections due to low white blood cell counts, bleeding due to low platelet counts, and even leukemia developing years later have been reported in patients receiving high doses of numerous drugs. Because more aggressive therapy will not necessarily produce more cures, some oncologists use less intensive treatment, particularly for elderly or very sick patients, in an effort to reduce complications.

Experimental programs for autologous marrow transplant (AMT) are attempting to reduce instances of low white blood cell counts or low platelet counts caused by high-dose chemotherapy. The technique involves obtaining bone marrow from the patient before starting treatment and freezing it. The marrow is then injected back into the patient during periods when the risk of low cell counts is the greatest. The goal of this procedure is to reduce the time during which the patient has low white blood cell and platelet counts (see Chapter 8).

Responses to chemotherapy in limited stage disease are often complete, with no sign of any remaining tumor, in about 45 to 75 percent of cases. Approximately 15 percent of patients with limited disease will still be disease-free at the end of two years. With extensive disease, complete responses occur in 20 to 30 percent of cases. Most patients with advanced disease, and those who do not respond to therapy for limited disease, die within one year, with perhaps 2 percent surviving to two years.

Mesotheliomas

Mesotheliomas are closely related to lung cancers and are caused by exposure to asbestos, usually in smokers. These tumors involve the pleura, the lining of the lung. Without treatment, the prognosis for these patients is poor. Surgery and radiotherapy are often used to relieve symptoms and, occasionally, to attempt to cure the disease. If these therapies fail, chemotherapy may be tried. Palliative treatment includes drugs such as cytoxan, adriamycin, methotrexate, 5-fluorouracil, and 5-azacytidine, often used in combination. Adriamycin is especially active against these tumors. However, responses are commonly incomplete and of short duration.

Mesothelioma, lung cancer, breast cancer, lymphomas, and many other cancers spread to the pleura and cause fluid to accumulate in the space between the chest wall and the lining of the lung. The fluid is thought to come from the liquid portion of blood leaked from blood vessels into the space between the pleura and the chest wall in response to the presence of cancer cells in the lining of the lung. This is called a pleural effusion. If caused by lymphomas, these pleural effusions respond to radiotherapy of the enlarged lymph glands in the chest and under the breastbone. Effusions caused by the other malignancies (mesothelioma, lung cancer, or breast cancer) are treated by injecting a drug into the space containing the fluid. The drug causes inflammation and scarring in the tissues lining the space and pastes them together, removing the space and squeezing out the fluid. The drug most commonly used for this purpose is tetracycline, an antibiotic.

Radioisotopes (radiophosphorus) and drugs such as quinacrine, adriamycin, and bleomycin are also used to treat pleural effusions. A tube is inserted into the pleural space through the chest wall to instill the drugs and to drain the space before and after treatment. The chest tube itself, or in combination with an injection of tetracycline, causes irritation of the lining, helping to close the space and eliminate fluid.

Fluid may accumulate in the abdomen as well as the pleura. These accumulations, called ascites, are difficult to treat if the tumor causing the condition fails to respond to therapy. Some of the drugs used for pleural effusions have been tried but are less effective when used to treat effusions in the abdomen. Thiotepa may be the best drug to date. Side effects include lowering of white cell, red cell, or platelet counts, but are otherwise not severe. Recently, devices known as shunts have been developed that channel fluid from the abdomen back into the bloodstream. These shunts are permanently implanted into the patient's body. This, of course, produces a risk of infection from its presence. Sometimes tumor cells clog the shunt, making it inoperative. Despite these complications, a shunt can relieve the discomfort and pain caused by ascites. Relief is possible even if the shunt only partially prevents the accumulation of fluid in the abdomen.

Ovarian Cancer

Mrs. C., a fifty-year-old woman in excellent physical condition, noticed that her abdomen was swollen and sought medical attention. Examination revealed a large mass filling her pelvis, and an ultrasound test detected fluid in her abdomen. Surgery was done to remove a large tumor originating in the ovary and several metastatic tumors on the membranes lining her abdomen. No visible tumor remained after the surgery. A blood test showed high levels of a substance called Ca 125, indicating that the tumor was still present. On advice of her oncologist, she received six cycles of alternating intravenous chemotherapy as soon as she recovered from surgery. She had a great deal of nausea and vomiting, suffered one serious infection, and lost most of her hair, which subsequently grew back. A second operation revealed no evidence of her cancer except for a few hard-to-identify cancer cells detected in random biopsy samples from membranes lining her abdomen and pelvis. Radiotherapy was directed to her abdomen over a period of six weeks, during which she again experienced nausea, vomiting, and extreme weakness. With difficulty, she tolerated the treatment and has not had a recurrence for five years.

The ovaries are the two glands in the female reproductive system that produce eggs, called ova, and certain hormones involved in reproductive functions. They are located inside the pelvic cavity, one on either side of the uterus. There are many types of ovarian tumors. The most common type is an adenocarcinoma of the ovary and, when oncologists speak about ovarian cancer, they are usually referring to this type. In the ovary are cells, like those in the bronchi and other organs, which secrete hormones. These cells may become cancerous, and the resulting tumor is called adenocarcinoma of the ovary. Cancers arising from other ovarian cells are rare (less than 10 percent of ovarian cancers) and are generally treatable or curable with surgery and radiotherapy. Chemotherapy plays some role in treating these unusual ovarian tumors, but because they are rare, their treatment is not described here.

Ovarian cancer of any type generally passes through four stages: (1) the ovarian stage (confined to the ovary); (2) the pelvic stage (limited to spread within the pelvis); (3) the peritoneal stage (spread to the lining of the pelvis and abdomen); and (4) the metastasized stage (spread outside the abdomen or pelvis to affect organs such as the liver and lung). Surgery and radiation are used to relieve and possibly cure disease confined to the ovary and pelvis; the more advanced stages are treated with surgery, followed by chemotherapy.

As with other tumors, such as colon and testicular disease, a marker protein usually exists in the blood of patients with advanced ovarian cancer. A marker is a substance that indicates, or marks, the presence of disease. In ovarian cancer, this protein, called Ca 125, is used to evaluate how the tumor responds to chemotherapy. As the tumor shrinks, the amount of Ca 125 in the blood declines; as it spreads, the protein concentration increases. Because Ca 125 is not always detectable in patients with ovarian cancer, its presence cannot be used to screen patients for diagnosis of the disease.

Abdominal surgery is performed to remove the ovary that contains the tumor. During the operation, the surgeon examines the area and takes biopsies to decide if other organs should be removed. Other adjacent organs such as the uterus and the ovary on the other side, or adjacent lymph nodes, are also removed if cancer cells are present or if there is a possibility that the cancer will spread to these areas. This procedure is called "debulking."

Current chemotherapy consists of three drugs given intravenously: cyclophosphamide, adriamycin, and cisplatin. The latter drug is considered the most effective and is usually administered in combination with one or both of the other drugs to treat patients with advanced ovarian cancer. Drugs are typically administered in four to six or more monthly cycles after surgery has been performed.

In certain cases an even more complex program is used. After drug therapy is completed and the Ca 125 level returns to normal, a second operation, a laparoscopy (an examination of the inside of the abdomen with a narrow bore instrument inserted through the abdominal wall), is performed to look for remaining tumor in the abdomen. If no tumor is found, even after the microscopic examination of the tissues and fluids removed, then chemotherapy can be stopped. Ten to 20 percent are cured. If more tumor is found or recurs, it may be removable. In any case, salvage chemotherapy with more toxic and generally less effective drugs can be administered in a last-ditch effort to destroy tumor cells not removable by surgery.

If the remaining tumor is visible only under a microscope, then radiotherapy may be directed to the entire abdomen, or more likely chemotherapy will be administered after the patient recovers from the second surgery. Patients who have had previous chemotherapy may experience nausea and vomiting, weakness, and infections as a result of radiotherapy to the entire abdomen. However, long-term survivals, probably cures, have been reported in patients with advanced ovarian cancers treated by this combined modality therapy.

Experimental trials are now under way that combine salvage therapy with implants of the patient's own bone marrow. If a patient has a relapse after surgery or standard chemotherapy, extremely high doses of cytoxan or other drugs may be required. At these high doses, the bone marrow is suppressed and unable to function. Bone marrow material is taken from the patient and frozen before chemotherapy begins. Later, when the blood cell levels fall as a result of the high-dose chemotherapy, the bone marrow is injected back into the patient, restoring her ability to produce blood cells.

While waiting for bone marrow function to return, patients receive blood transfusions to restore blood volume quickly and antibiotics to fight off infections (see Chapter 8).

Unfortunately most patients with ovarian cancer do not do as well as Mrs. C. Her case is important, however, because many patients undergo this sort of treatment even though the ultimate outlook is poor. If their disease is further advanced, the surgeon cannot remove enough of the tumor, or the residual tumor resists chemotherapy. Therefore, for the vast majority of patients, chemotherapy is given to relieve pain, to remove blockage of the intestines, or to decrease accumulation of fluid in the abdomen. No single combination of drugs is accepted by all oncologists as first-line, initial therapy. Most agree that a drug called cisplatin is the most effective and that it should be given in combination with either cyclophosphamide, adriamycin, or both. Since cisplatin has adverse effects on the kidneys, patients with kidney failure are treated with one of the other two drugs.

Very recently, carboplatin (Parplatin) has been approved by the FDA for the treatment of patients with ovarian cancer. It is related chemically to cisplatin and may be used as a substitute for it. This drug causes less vomiting and less damage to the kidneys, hearing, and nervous system than cisplatin. It is not more effective than cisplatin, however, and it can cause a greater degree of bone marrow suppression. This can result in a greater risk of infection or bleeding for the patient, due to low white cell and platelet counts. Although its exact role in treating ovarian cancer has not yet been determined, oncologists may well include carboplatin in programs to treat this disease.

Many patients, especially those who are elderly and frail, cannot tolerate combination therapy. For these patients oral medications, such as chlorambucil, or phenylalanine mustard, or cyclophosphamide, are given to relieve symptoms.

Several new techniques and drugs are currently under investigation for treatment of ovarian cancer. Researchers have identified a growth modifier, called Mullerian-inhibiting substance, found in embryos, which inhibits the growth of ovarian cancer cells grown in the laboratory. Perhaps some day such naturally occurring material will be used to treat this disease without the toxic side effects of current treatments.

Immunotherapy is another technique that is being investigated. Immunotherapy uses the body's own immune system to attack cancer cells. In general terms, the immune system consists of cells that make chemicals called antibodies. Antibodies are initially produced when a substance not normally found in the body, called an antigen, gets in. When the antigen again enters the body, the antibodies attack it with a great deal of power and selectivity. Modern-day genetic engineering processes have enabled scientists to produce antibodies in the laboratory. Although they have been unsuccessful so far, these so-called monoclonal antibodies are being developed to deliver drugs to the tumor or to destroy the cancer cells directly.

Another experimental approach places drugs into the abdomen through a tube. High concentrations of anticancer drugs then bathe the cancer cells that adhere to the lining of the abdomen. Cancers that resist usual concentrations of the drugs may respond to these much higher doses. More clinical work needs to be done to determine whether this approach is beneficial and whether patients can tolerate its side effects.

It is very difficult to determine the prognosis for individual patients with advanced ovarian cancer. Much of the outcome depends on how much tumor can be removed at the time of surgery and whether the tumor is considered of high- or low-grade malignancy. A high-grade malignancy is one that is more likely to spread quickly, reducing survival time. A small percentage of patients (3 to 5 percent) with advanced cancer can be cured by surgery and chemotherapy, but most cannot be. Many more, perhaps 40 to 60 percent, will experience less pain and an improvement in activity level with the combined treatments. With skillful chemotherapy, some patients may live for one or two years. As with other cancers, more powerful drugs with fewer side effects are needed if there is to be significant improvement in cure rates. In any case, some sort of modern chemotherapy can and should be administered to almost all patients with advanced ovarian cancer. It may improve the quality of life, and there is always a chance that a patient may go into complete remission and remain there for years.

Skin Cancer

Skin, the external covering of the body, is actually an organ, just like the heart, liver, lungs, or ovaries. It is made up of a number of cell layers, any of which may become cancerous. Skin cancer is the most common malignancy. It is also the most easily cured, usually by surgery. Some skin cancers, such as basal cell, which involves the skin's inner layer, and squamous cell, which involves the outer layer, also respond to radiation. With rare exception, chemotherapy plays no role in initial treatment of skin cancer. Chemotherapy does play a role, however, in treating two relatively rare types of skin cancer, namely melanoma and Kaposi's sarcoma.

Malignant Melanoma

A melanoma is a pigmented mole or tumor of the skin. Malignant melanoma is a type of cancer that must be cured by surgery, if it can be cured at all. Substantial research has gone into finding drugs that might cure or at least relieve melanoma that has spread or is otherwise unlikely to be cured by surgery. So far, the results have been disappointing. Responses have been seen, but they are generally limited to short-lived regression of tumor in skin and lymph glands. Once the disease has spread, as it often does, to the liver, bones, lungs, or brain, it is essentially incurable and will not respond to chemotherapy. Immunomodulators, a new class of drugs including interferon and interleukin-2, are being investigated but, so far, have had only limited success. However, I urge patients with advanced disease to seek out this therapy.

Dacarbazine is a drug that has been extensively studied for the treatment of malignant melanoma that cannot be cured with surgery. It is severely toxic to the gastrointestinal system, causing nausea and vomiting. Various dosing schedules, routes of administration, and combined therapies have been attempted, but it has not yet cured, or even controlled, such cases. Occasionally responses are seen. However, no better nonexperimental therapy exists.

Kaposi's Sarcoma

This is a rare but treatable form of skin cancer now being diagnosed more frequently because of its association with AIDS (ac-
quired immune deficiency syndrome). In the past, this cancer was
seen without evidence of AIDS. Skin lesions, or ulcers, usually
appear on the legs before progressing slowly to other parts of the
skin. These lesions may cause pain or cosmetic disfigurement, for
example, if they are on the face, or they may ulcerate and become
infected. The lesions can also infiltrate into body organs, causing
pain and interfering with normal function. Patients ultimately die
when other organs, such as the lymph nodes, become involved
or when infections develop because of AIDS itself or its treatment.

Treatment includes various forms of radiation such as electron
beams and X rays to the skin and deeper organs, but most patients
require chemotherapy. Vinblastine chemotherapy given by vein
once a week causes some improvement by reducing the size and
number of lesions and remains the primary drug for treatment of
this cancer. However, trials are under way with vinblastine, dacti-
nomycin, cyclophosphamide, vincristine, dacarbazine, carmustine,
bleomycin, and adriamycin used either singly or in combination. These drugs may yield better results by increasing the number of patients who benefit, particularly in advanced stages of the
disease.

Head and Neck Cancer

Cancers of the lips, mouth, pharynx, larynx, nose, sinuses, ear, and
salivary glands are usually grouped together as cancers of the head
and neck. Surgery and radiotherapy are the mainstays of therapy
for these cancers. Chemotherapy is used almost exclusively in patients with tumors too advanced to be cured by these methods or
those who have relapsed following treatment. Squamous cell can-

cers are the most frequent form of head and neck cancer. Symptoms are generally relieved by chemotherapy with several different drugs, often used in combination or one after the other. (Treatment of lymphomas and sarcomas in the head and neck was discussed in Chapter 5.)

The major difficulty with these cancers is that they cannot be cured once surgery and radiation have failed. Most tumors—about 75 percent—respond to chemotherapy, but they almost always return and become resistant to further treatment. Some 10 to 15 percent of patients will reach complete remission, but for only an average of less than one year. Because side effects are tolerable, chemotherapy is almost always useful in relieving symptoms, but no standard program exists. Oncologists usually rely on methotrexate, cisplatin, 5-fluorouracil, bleomycin, and vinblastine, in any combination, although there is little firm evidence that a particular combination is better than methotrexate alone for initial chemotherapy. Cisplatin, bleomycin, and methotrexate have been administered into arteries supplying blood to the cancers and also by continuous infusion into a vein, with unconfirmed reports of better results by the latter technique. In some cases, the tumor regresses enough to allow surgical removal and perhaps long-term disease-free survival.

Treatment programs vary widely both in terms of the number of drugs used and dosing schedules. Methotrexate is often given by vein once every two or three weeks, bleomycin by vein or muscle twice a week, and cisplatin by vein daily for five days every three weeks. There are many side effects, including painful mouth ulcers, called mucositis, and potential kidney damage. If radiation therapy is given along with these drugs, the mouth ulcers will often be significantly worse.

Few cancers require as much planning for therapy as these do. Ideally, initial treatment should involve a team of surgeons who are experts in head and neck operations, radiation oncologists with experience using computers and modern radiation equipment, and medical oncologists with interest in this type of cancer. Physicians and equipment such as this are available at cancer treatment centers throughout the United States.

Cancer of the Prostate

The prostate gland surrounds the neck of the bladder and the urethra in the male. It produces a thin fluid that becomes part of semen. A prostate tumor can block the urethra, preventing urination. Surgery is used to remove the obstruction and the prostate gland itself. In some early cases, radiotherapy alone can relieve obstruction and successfully treat the cancer. Fortunately, surgery and radiation are effective therapy for early disease.

If surgery or radiation is not successful and the patient has symptoms requiring treatment, hormonal therapy is usually begun. Four types of treatment are available, all of which interfere with or reduce levels of testosterone, a hormone that cancer cells may need to live and proliferate. Removal of the testes, which make testosterone, is one method. Although the surgery results in impotence and infertility, it relieves pain from tumor spreading to the bones and it can keep symptoms under control for years.

Equally effective is hormonal treatment with female sex hormones, estrogens. Estrogens suppress the pituitary gland at the base of the brain. The pituitary gland produces a number of hormones and other chemicals that regulate many bodily processes, including factors that stimulate testosterone production. As therapy, however, estrogens cause the patient's body to become feminized by taking on some female characteristics, and they are associated with cardiovascular complications, including heart attacks and heart failure.

To overcome this problem, researchers developed a third hormonal strategy. Daily injections of a synthetic hormone, leuprolide, are used to inhibit the pituitary gland. Inhibiting the pituitary with leuprolide yields the same results as the other two strategies without surgery and without side effects caused by estrogen. However, daily injections are required and the drug is expensive, approximately $400 per month.

Recently a fourth hormonal approach to controlling advanced prostate cancer has become available. Flutamide (Eulexin), an oral antiandrogen drug, has shown activity against this cancer. The drug interferes with the activity of all androgens—that is, male hormones in general, including testosterone. Flutamide may be considered for patients who use leuprolide.

Because chemotherapy has limited success in prostate cancer, it is used only after radiotherapy and hormonal therapy have failed. Chemotherapy for cancer of the prostate gland is in its infancy. So far, no single drug has been sufficiently effective against this tumor to warrant combining it with other drugs, hormones, or radiation to improve survival. One interesting drug is estramustine, which combines estrogen with a compound similar to nitrogen mustard. Doctors hoped that the estrogen part of the drug would attach to receptors on the cancer cells, allowing the anticancer part to kill the cells. Unfortunately, the success rate for this drug is no better or worse than others. Other drugs used alone or in combination include FAM (5-fluorouracil, adriamycin, and mitomycin C), cyclophosphamide, and methotrexate. Only 15 percent of patients with advanced prostate cancer will gain relief from pain from chemotherapy.

Kidney and Bladder Cancers

The kidneys are two organs located at the back of the abdominal cavity, one on each side of the backbone. They remove waste material from the blood and excrete it as urine into the bladder. The bladder then acts as a reservoir, collecting urine and discharging it into the urethra for elimination from the body.

Kidney Cancer

No useful chemotherapy exists for kidney cancer. Surgical removal is the only hope of cure. Standard chemotherapy does not even relieve symptoms of this disease. Surgical removal is often performed to prevent or reduce bleeding, pain, and infection even when a cure is not possible. Spontaneous remissions sometimes occur, but they may not last long. Recently, some hope has been aroused by immunomodulating drugs, such as interferon and interleukin, which enhance the body's own defenses against cancer cells. It remains to be seen whether this class of drugs will finally give some hope to patients with kidney cancer. Patients should seriously consider entering experimental trials that use these drugs.

Bladder Cancer

In bladder cancer, as in kidney cancer, chemotherapy plays a very limited role. Chemotherapy is considered only when surgery and radiation have not been effective. Many drugs have been tried, but few patients experience pain relief completely even when the drugs are used in combination. Bleomycin, cisplatin, cyclophosphamide, and adriamycin are among the more active drugs used in the treatment of this disease. Two other drugs, methotrexate and vinblastine, have been combined with cisplatin and adriamycin in a program called M-VAC. This combination can give some complete remissions (36 percent), but unfortunately most patients receiving this treatment have relapsed, and only a relative few have survived long-term.

Bladder cancer sometimes involves only the superficial lining of the organ—this is referred to as superficial bladder cancer. This type of tumor can be treated with chemotherapy instilled, or slowly dripped, into the bladder with a catheter or an instrument called a cystoscope. A cystoscope is an instrument that consists of a tube with a bright light on one end. The tip farthest from the light source is passed through the outer opening of the urethra into the bladder. The physician turns on the light, which travels through optical fibers in the tube to illuminate the area inside the patient's bladder. The physician can then examine the bladder, urethra, and, in male patients, part of the prostate gland through which the urethra passes. The cystoscope can also be used to remove or destroy cancerous tumors on the lining of the bladder, or to open up the urethra if it is blocked because the prostate gland is enlarged.

Thiotepa and adriamycin are two drugs used successfully to treat this cancer. Multiple instillations are often required, and it is necessary to monitor carefully for spread of the cancer into the bladder wall. If it does spread, the patient must undergo surgical removal of all or part of the bladder. Recently, interferon has been used alone or in combination with other drugs to treat this fairly common malignancy. Initial reports are encouraging and side effects are few, usually consisting of fever, malaise, and chills.

Another experimental approach to treating superficial bladder cancer is to inject hematin, a drug that is taken up only by cancer cells. The bladder lining is then exposed to intense light. Hematin in the cancer cells, when exposed to this light, responds by forming a chemical that destroys the cancer cells. The major side effect is irritation of the bladder, causing pain or bleeding during urination.

Bone Cancer and Related Diseases

Multiple Myeloma

Mr. W. developed rib fractures and bone pain following a minor injury. His physician found that he was anemic, and a bone marrow examination revealed the presence of myeloma plasma cells. Large quantities of immunoglobulin proteins were present in his urine and serum. Bone X rays revealed bone deterioration in his ribs, spine, and skull. His oncologist found that, despite widespread myeloma, Mr. W. had normal kidney function and no complications. Oral doses of phenylalanine mustard and prednisone given every six weeks reduced his production of immunoglobulins and completely relieved his bone pain. His fractures healed, and he had no subsequent fractures for five years.

Unfortunately, after five years his ribs again became painful and his protein levels rose. He also showed evidence of kidney failure and developed a bleeding problem because of a low platelet count. All this occurred despite continued therapy with phenylalanine mustard and prednisone. His oncologist chose to discontinue these drugs and started using dexamethasone. Slowly, he felt better; his protein levels fell toward normal and kidney function improved somewhat. He required frequent transfusions of platelets and red cells during this time. Finally he stabilized and, with intermittent dexamethasone treatments, lived a relatively normal life for one year.

Next, he had a bout of bleeding from a large stomach ulcer caused by the dexamethasone. This occurred despite drug therapy aimed at preventing stomach ulcers from forming. The bleeding complicated his persistent kidney failure, and he required kidney dialysis. Dialysis is a procedure for treating the patient's blood to remove liquids and chemicals normally removed by the kidneys. A final, fatal complication was an infection, carried in the bloodstream, which probably started in his kidneys. Altogether, he lived for six and one-half years after his cancer was diagnosed and for most of that time was able to function at home and at work.

Multiple myeloma is often referred to as "bone cancer." It is actually a malignancy of the bone marrow rather than the bones themselves. Bone marrow is located inside certain adult bones and is the place where blood cells—red cells, white cells, and platelets—are produced. Most of the marrow in the body is contained in the spine, breastbone, ribs, and pelvic or hip bones. One type of normal marrow cell is called the plasma cell. Malignant proliferation of these cells produces a type of tumor called a myeloma. Because these tumors form at a number of sites within the marrow, the disease is called multiple myeloma. The disease is accompanied by plasma cells in the bloodstream; high levels of immunoglobulins—proteins (actually antibodies) made by plasma cells; anemia due to interference with red cell production; bone pain; and kidney damage. Although the disease is incurable, many patients are relieved of symptoms for years with chemotherapy.

The amount of bone involved and number of complications determine, to a large extent, which chemotherapy is used. Patients with uncomplicated myeloma—no kidney damage, no high blood calcium, no severe anemia—are treated with phenylalanine mustard, a drug similar to chlorambucil and cyclophosphamide, in combination with synthetic adrenal corticosteroids, such as prednisone. Several programs exist for administering phenylalanine mustard, which is taken orally. Daily or alternate-day doses are prescribed with close attention to monitoring the patient's white blood cell count. Because phenylalanine mustard's effect on white cell counts is often delayed for days or weeks, the dose must be promptly reduced at the first sign of a falling white cell count, to prevent low counts and reduce the risk of infection.

Another program used for patients with myeloma also employs phenylalanine mustard along with prednisone. Doses are given orally for four to seven consecutive days and repeated every four to six weeks, modified according to white blood cell counts. Beneficial effects of both programs include control of bone pain, decrease in the amount of abnormal blood protein, stabilization of red cell counts, and improvement in kidney function.

Multiple myeloma patients with more advanced disease can suffer complications including kidney failure, high blood calcium from bone loss, high levels of the abnormal immunoglobulins, extensive bone damage or fractures, and severe anemia. A number of programs are available for these patients. Cyclophosphamide, phenylalanine mustard, vincristine, carmustine, and corticosteroids are used in various combinations or all together, as in the so-called M-2 protocol. These combinations are more likely to benefit a patient with advanced disease than the two-drug program using phenylalanine mustard and prednisone. Adriamycin is another drug used in combinations for the treatment of myeloma. This multiple-drug chemotherapy causes a number of side effects that complicate the lives of myeloma patients, with infection, bleeding, hair loss, anemia, mouth sores, and vomiting heading the list.

About 70 percent of myeloma patients achieve symptom relief with chemotherapy. Virtually all experience relief from pain, and some show improvement in appetite, kidney function, and mobility, as well as fewer bone fractures. Patients receiving chemotherapy can increase their life expectancy, on average, by about two years. It is very difficult to make predictions about life span for an individual patient. Some patients have a surprisingly long clinical remission and life span, while others succumb early to their disease. With chemotherapy, a patient with early-stage disease may expect to live approximately four years and a patient with advanced disease, two to three years. These are twice the life expectancies of patients who do not receive chemotherapy.

A number of patients with less advanced disease become stabilized after twenty-four months of treatment, and immunoglobulin levels fall and remain low. These patients may be taken off drug therapy with the expectation that they will stay in remission. This drug holiday, as it is called, probably reduces phenylalanine mustard's leukemogenic potential, that is, it becomes less likely to cause leukemia after two or more years of therapy. The patient and physician should consider this very carefully, however, because doctors have only limited experience with stopping treatment, and there is always the risk that a patient may relapse and not respond to further therapy. Obviously, if the disease progresses, treatment must be started again quickly.

Recently a study was done of the beneficial effects of a myeloma program that included adriamycin, vincristine, and the adrenal corticosteroid dexamethasone. During the study, investigators were surprised to learn that huge doses of oral dexamethasone alone, in cycles, was effective therapy. In fact, many patients, especially those with less advanced disease and those who had failed to respond to multiple-agent chemotherapy, received the most benefit from this program. Large daily doses of dexamethasone are given cyclically then no drug is given for two weeks. This cycling is repeated indefinitely if the patient's symptoms improve and abnormal immunoglobulins decrease.

Despite chemotherapy, most myeloma patients ultimately die from infections or kidney failure. Radiotherapy is sometimes used to treat painful lesions in the bone or tumors that spread to the spinal cord. Immunomodulators such as interferon are being tried experimentally with some success, as mentioned in Chapter 5. Also, autologous bone marrow transplantation, a procedure similar to that used to treat non-Hodgkin's lymphoma, is being investigated (see Chapter 8).

Waldenstrom's Macroglobulinemia

This disease is closely related to multiple myeloma. It is characterized by the presence of large-size proteins in the bloodstream and abnormal lymphocytes in the bone marrow. The disease usually progresses very slowly, and treatment begins only when symptoms occur or seem likely to begin. Standard treatment is daily oral doses of chlorambucil. Patients with advanced or progressive disease obtain symptom relief with treatment programs similar to those used to treat multiple myeloma.

Sarcomas

Sarcomas are rare cancers of the body's supporting tissues, such as muscle or bone. There are two types of tumors, one affecting the hard, supporting substance of bones—these are not cancers that spread to the bones or originate in the bone marrow, as myeloma does—and soft tissue sarcomas. Soft tissue sarcomas start in muscle, fat, fibrous tissue, blood vessels, nerves, and other supporting tissues of the body. For treatment purposes, they are divided into tumors involving the arms and legs and those involving the rest of the body.

Sarcomas are usually treated first with surgery and radiotherapy. In these cases, chemotherapy is used as additive therapy. Additive chemotherapy is intended to aid the effectiveness of surgery and radiation by destroying cancer cells. Chemotherapy is also used as palliative therapy to relieve symptoms for some sarcomas. Since these tumors are rare and the exact role of chemotherapy is uncertain for this disease, it is best to begin therapy in a cancer center equipped with an experienced team of surgical, radiation, and medical oncologists.

Sarcomas of the Bone

Osteogenic sarcoma and Ewing's sarcoma affect the bones and are often treated with additive chemotherapy along with surgery and radiation. The goal is to reduce the amount of surgery required for cure and to try to prevent the disease from spreading. Such therapy uses multiple combinations of drugs such as vincristine, adriamycin, methotrexate, cisplatin, bleomycin, actinomycin D, or cyclophosphamide. There are still no standard guidelines to administering these drugs and choosing a treatment program. It does appear, however, that chemotherapy has spared many patients from limb amputation and enabled cures with less extensive surgery than would otherwise have been required.

Soft Tissue Sarcomas of the Arms and Legs

In adults, these sarcomas are treated in a manner similar to bone sarcomas. Limb-sparing surgery, radiation, and additive chemotherapy often produce disease-free survival. Adriamycin, cyclophosphamide, and methotrexate are commonly used. Often, as with bone sarcomas, high doses of methotrexate require use of an antidote, leucovorin, to prevent severe toxicity. The patient receives an infusion of methotrexate. Then, twenty-four hours later, doses of the antidote are taken orally. The twenty-four-hour intervening period is when the drug attacks the cancer cells. Unfortunately this drug also affects normal cells, and serious side effects result if the normal cells are exposed for longer than twenty-four hours. Side effects include diarrhea, vomiting, infections, bleeding, and kidney failure. The antidote reduces toxicity to normal cells, particularly in the intestines and mouth. Doctors must closely monitor the methotrexate levels in the blood and function of the kidneys during this procedure, especially when higher doses of methotrexate are used.

Soft Tissue Sarcomas of the Adult Trunk

These sarcomas do not respond to treatment as well as those of the extremities. Investigational studies are being done using dacarbazine, adriamycin, cyclophosphamide, and a related drug, ifosfamide. Actinomycin D and vincristine have also been used. Although chemotherapy does not usually cure the disease, it can stabilize and relieve symptoms for some patients.

Soft Tissue Sarcomas in Children

These sarcomas may be cured using combined surgery, radiation, and chemotherapy. A 60 percent cure rate has been reported in these cases. Embryonal rhabdomyosarcoma, a tumor of skeletal muscle, is the most common type of soft tissue sarcoma, and chemotherapy has been successful in its treatment. Treatment of this tumor and retinoblastoma, tumor of the eye, is individualized, requiring specialized and complex care by pediatric oncologists.

Cancer of the Liver and Bile Ducts

The liver is the largest organ in the body. It is located in the right side, below the diaphragm separating the abdomen from the chest cavity. The liver has many functions involved with digestion, waste removal, blood cell circulation, blood clotting, and manufacture and storage of important substances. One of these substances, called bile, is made in the liver; it passes into the gallbladder for storage or flows directly into the small intestine, where it breaks down fats as part of the digestive process. The structures through which the bile passes are called bile ducts. Cancer may start in the lining of the bile ducts and obstruct them, or cancers present in the liver can obstruct the openings into the bile ducts.

Cancer Arising from Liver Cells

Cancer can spread to the liver from abdominal organs, such as the colon or pancreas, or from almost any other area of the body. Two types of cancers, however, arise directly from liver cells. One is called a hepatoma and the other is cancer of the bile ducts. These conditions are quite rare in the United States but occur frequently in the Orient. We do not know why these two cancers are more common in the Orient, but it may be related to the large number of patients with liver parasites or hepatitis in that part of the world. The tumors originate in cells contained only in the liver and its ducts, passageways leading out of the liver. They are usually incurable at the time of diagnosis, although early surgery to remove part of the liver will sometimes cure the disease. Such surgery is successful only if no residual tumor is left behind. Radiation therapy or chemotherapy is often required to relieve pain, accumulation of fluid in the abdomen, or vomiting.

Unfortunately, few drugs have any effect on these tumors. Adriamycin, methotrexate, and 5-fluorouracil injected by vein or given directly into the blood supply to the liver have been tried but with little long-term success. These drugs are probably worth trying, however, if the patient has pain and jaundice (yellowing of the skin and other tissues due to accumulated bile pigments). Unless the disease is cured surgically, chemotherapy will give only short-term relief of pain and jaundice.

Techniques have been suggested to cut off the blood supply to these tumors to relieve symptoms. By cutting off blood supply, some part of the tumor will die from lack of oxygen. There is little hazard, except pain from death of the tumor tissue. The main problem is that any relief from pain is usually short-lived, because the tumors rapidly grow back to their original size or even larger. One pain-relieving, strictly palliative, procedure is to surgically close off arteries supplying blood to the tumor. The other involves inserting a catheter into these arteries and injecting materials designed to block the flow of blood.

Stomach and Esophageal Cancer

The stomach and the esophagus are organs of the gastrointestinal, or digestive, tract. As with other tumors of the gastrointestinal tract, the only therapy that can cure stomach or esophageal cancer is surgical removal before the tumor spreads to other areas. Radiotherapy is used for symptom relief in patients undergoing surgery. Palliative chemotherapy may be given to patients with no hope of surgical cure who have or are likely to develop painful symptoms. The usual symptoms are pain and vomiting from obstruction of the upper gastrointestinal tract, resulting in weight loss. There is no clear evidence, however, that such chemotherapy prolongs life or even actually relieves symptoms. Some patients die earlier than expected from the effects of treatment, and some experience worse symptoms because of side effects. For these reasons, it is often difficult for patients and oncologists to decide if and when chemotherapy should be given for this disease. In this situation, no therapy may be the best solution.

Doctors often employ FAM treatment (5-fluorouracil, adriamycin, and mitomycin-C), which involves administering all three drugs by vein in cycles repeated every three weeks. Another program (APE) combines adriamycin, cisplatin, and etoposide. All too frequently there is no response, and some side effects occur. Side effects associated with these drugs commonly include infections, bleeding, gastrointestinal symptoms, hair loss, and heart problems. Programs using chemotherapy with surgery or radiation are also used for symptom relief.

Cancer of the Pancreas

The pancreas is a gland behind the stomach that connects with the upper part of the small intestine. Its primary function is to produce the hormones insulin and glucagon, substances that play a primary role in regulating storage and use of glucose, a type of sugar formed during digestion. The pancreas also produces enzymes necessary for normal digestion.

There is no useful chemotherapy for cancer of the pancreas. All attempts to use chemotherapy, even for symptom relief, have failed miserably. If surgical removal is incomplete or if the tumor returns after surgery, the patient will die. All that can be done is to relieve symptoms with radiation and narcotics, and to remove abdominal fluid that often accumulates in patients with advanced disease.

Physicians have recently become interested in treating pancreatic cancer with the combination of adriamycin, cisplatin, and etoposide or with the combination of 5FU given with leucovorin, the antidote used with high-dose methotrexate therapy. Apparently, leucovorin affects the metabolism of the vitamin folic acid in such a way that it enhances the antitumor effect of 5FU. More clinical studies are needed to confirm any long-term benefit of these two drug combinations.

A very rare malignancy of the pancreas, called islet cell tumor, causes hypoglycemia, which is a lowering of the blood sugar to levels where the patient has a seizure or becomes unconscious. The low blood sugar is because of excess production of insulin, a normal pancreatic secretion, from the tumor. Surgical removal of the tumor is the only hope for a cure. Unlike more common pancreatic cancers, symptoms from this tumor can be relieved with a drug called streptozotocin, administered by vein for five consecutive days every six weeks. Treatment is monitored by blood tests. Increased blood sugar and decreased insulin levels are evidence that the tumor is responding, while low white blood cell counts indicate bone marrow suppression, a side effect of the drug.

Blood Cell Cancers

One group of cancers results from uncontrolled proliferation of blood cells. Called myeloproliferative diseases, they affect the bone marrow, resulting in malignant overproduction of one or more of the cellular components of blood, namely white blood cells, red blood cells, and platelets. Diseases usually listed as myeloproliferative diseases include the following:

1. polycythemia vera, an overproduction of red blood cells
2. agnogenic myeloid metaplasia, a development of scar tissue in the bone marrow, affecting cell development
3. thrombocythemia, an overproduction of platelets
4. chronic myelocytic leukemia.

Chemotherapy is used to suppress bone marrow function and, therefore, lower blood cell counts toward a normal level. Removal of blood from a vein, called phlebotomy, is often used to lower red cell counts. Drugs used include cyclophosphamide, chlorambucil, busulfan, and radioactive phosphorus. The latter drug is a radioactive substance injected intravenously or taken orally. The drug then makes its way into the bloodstream. Blood bathes the bone marrow, allowing the radiation to enter sensitive cells within it, destroying their ability to make red cells, white cells, and platelets. The other three drugs prevent the bone marrow from producing cells. Unfortunately, chemotherapy treatment can lead to leukemia, but the risk is still there for those who receive no treatment. Researchers do not know why chemotherapy may in some cases increase the risk of developing leukemia. The reason may be related to the effect the treatment has on the metabolism of DNA, the cellular substance that is the chemical basis of heredity and genetic reproduction. Recently, fears of causing leukemia have encouraged the use of a drug called hydroxyurea. So far, this drug appears effective in suppressing bone marrow function with less risk than the other drugs for causing leukemia.

Except for radioactive phosphorus, which is administered intravenously or orally, the drugs are given orally as a daily dose. Effects on the bone marrow may take days or weeks, making it necessary to adjust doses frequently before establishing a stable maintenance dose. Drug holidays of weeks or months are often necessary to prevent permanent bone marrow damage or to allow symptoms to dissipate. (A drug holiday is a period of time when the patient does not take any drugs for the disease.)

Side effects from these drugs include infection caused, in part, by lowered white cell counts; bleeding due to low platelet counts; hair loss; nausea; and vomiting. Usually there are few or no side effects, and the patient is asymptomatic. When malignant blood cells die, they produce uric acid, an excess of which can damage the kidneys. Therefore, when the patient's white cell counts or blood uric acid levels are high, treatment with drugs such as allopurinol, which lower uric acid levels, helps prevent kidney damage.

Cancer of the Uterus

The uterus is the organ of the female reproductive system that contains and nourishes the embryo and fetus from the time of fertilization to the time of birth. Cancer of the uterus occurs at the mouth of the uterus, called the cervix, or in the lining of the organ, called the endometrium.

Cancer of the Cervix

Cervical cancer may be diagnosed at a very early stage by use of Pap smears, microscopic studies of cells collected from the cervix and vagina during a pelvic examination. If found in early stages, cervical cancer is curable with radiation, surgery, or both. For this reason, advanced cervical cancer is rare. If the disease is advanced, however, and incurable with surgery or radiotherapy, chemotherapy can relieve some of the uncomfortable symptoms of advanced disease. Symptoms include pain in the abdomen and pelvis, inability to defecate or urinate because the tumor obstructs the colon or outflow tracts from kidneys, fever, foul-smelling hard-to-treat infections in the pelvis and uterus, general malaise, and bleeding from ulcerated metastatic tumors. Bleomycin, methotrexate, and cisplatin are some of the drugs used. Unfortunately, any response in patients with advanced disease is generally short-lived, and they quickly succumb.

Cancer of the Endometrium

Cancer may begin in the lining of the uterus, which is called the endometrium. The initial symptom is often abnormal bleeding from the uterus, months or years after the patient's normal periods have stopped as part of menopause. The patient's uterus enlarges, and the cancer can be detected when the physician does a pelvic examination. Diagnosis is confirmed by a D&C, a surgical procedure. Under anesthesia, a surgeon scrapes the lining of the uterus and examines it under the microscope. If the cancer is discovered early, when it is present only in the endometrium, a patient has at least a 90 percent chance of cure by surgical removal of the uterus. If the tumor has spread outside the uterus and adjacent lymph nodes, however, the cure rate falls considerably. If it has spread into the pelvis or abdomen, it is uniformly fatal.

This disease is also curable in early stages by surgery and radiation. Once it has spread outside the uterus and associated lymph glands, however, the prognosis becomes poor. Hormones such as progesterones may bring relief when the disease spreads to the pelvis or lung. However, responses are incomplete and short-lasting. Adriamycin, used by itself or in combination with other drugs, such as cytoxan or cisplatin, has had some effect against these metastatic tumors, but response is no better than that obtained with hormones. Doctors often rely on radiotherapy to relieve symptoms that are the result of tumors that have spread to the pelvis, abdomen, or brain.

Brain Tumors

The brain consists of nerve tissue, enclosed within the upper part of the skull. It is a primary organ of the central nervous system, which is made up of the brain and the spinal cord. Malignant brain tumors that cannot be cured by surgery are usually treated with radiotherapy. If neither treatment is successful, little else can be done to cure the disease. Many attempts have been made to cure common brain tumors, called gliomas, with a drug called carmustine. Its side effects include nausea, vomiting, hair loss, infections because of low white blood cell counts, and bleeding because of low platelet counts. Unfortunately, there seems to be little benefit from its use. Other drugs that have been used with varying degrees of success are vincristine, methotrexate, and procarbazine. Immunomodulators, such as interferon, are being tested against these hard-to-treat tumors. Doctors usually encourage patients who are in need of symptom relief for brain tumors to try experimental therapies.

Immunotherapy

Recent approaches to chemotherapy are intended to stimulate the patient's own defenses to rid the body of cancers. Animal studies show that tumors can be cured when the body sees the cancer cells as foreign and produces natural chemicals to attack them. Results in humans, however, have been disappointing thus far. Nevertheless, some approaches deserve consideration, particularly in patients whose disease resists standard treatment or where no effective therapy exists. Research in this field is intense, and enthusiasm grows or diminishes along with varying reports of success or failure. Except for the treatment that employs a drug called alpha interferon, immunotherapy can be administered only through a clinical trial. Indicated use and treatment schedules are changing rapidly for this emerging group of immunotherapy drugs. Therefore, I'll briefly discuss only a few of the drugs.

Interferons

These drugs are made by cells naturally in response to exposure to viruses and other foreign substances. They appear actually to destroy cancer cells. Only one type, alpha interferon, has been approved by the FDA. It is used to treat a rare type of leukemia called hairy cell leukemia and Kaposi's sarcoma, a malignancy of the skin often seen in patients with AIDS (see Chapters 5 and 6). The patient self-administers the drug by injection as often as three times a week. Common side effects include fever, chills, muscle aches, fatigue, reduced appetite, and lowered white blood cell counts. Partial symptom relief has been reported in other malignancies treated with interferon, including lymphomas, kidney tumors, melanoma, myeloma, chronic myelocytic leukemia, bladder cancer, and carcinoid tumor. Researchers have yet to determine the real effectiveness of interferons. So far, other types of interferon are no more effective against cancer than alpha interferon.

Monoclonal Antibodies

These drugs are under intense evaluation for their usefulness in the treatment of cancer. Antibodies are substances produced in response to the presence of certain proteins called antigens. The antibodies attack the patient's tumor cells, inactivating or destroying them. The body naturally produces a small quantity of antibodies, but laboratory technology has made possible large-scale production of monoclonal antibodies.

One use of monoclonal antibodies is employing them to carry standard chemotherapy to malignant cells. Because they are specifically drawn to the cells of the tumor, they can bring the chemotherapy directly to only the tumor cells. Monoclonal antibodies, some chemically attached to chemotherapeutic drugs, are being studied for activity in leukemias, lymphomas, myeloma, melanoma, and cancers of the stomach, brain, liver, breast, and colon.

Unfortunately, the overall results of monoclonal antibody therapy have been disappointing. So far such treatment has been unsuccessful, because the antigens located on tumors seem to change with time and become unaffected by chemotherapy. In some cases, the antigen on the surface of the patient's tumor cells is eventually removed, making the cancer cells unresponsive to the effect of the antibody. The treatment is totally experimental and as yet has no practical use.

Monoclonal antibodies have been used to "clean up" previously stored bone marrow before it is injected back into the patient (see Chapter 8). The monoclonal antibodies help destroy any remaining cancer cells. The best results with this technique have been seen in the treatment of lymphomas. Lymphoma patients are treated with large amounts of radiotherapy or chemotherapy to destroy the cancer cells. This intense therapy causes severe suppression of the bone marrow, increasing the likelihood of bleeding and infection. After cleaning by antibodies, the patient's returned marrow is both functional and free of cancer cells.

Interleukin-2 (IL-2)

This drug is called a lymphokine because it is naturally produced by human lymphocytes, a type of white blood cell. It has a number of effects on the body's immune system and responds in many ways to cancer cells. When combined with special white blood cells called killer lymphocytes or lymphokine activated killer cells (LAK cells), IL-2 has produced symptom relief in melanoma and cancers of the lung, kidney, breast, and colon. Still, the treatment does not cure these tumors, and some studies have reported that these treatments cause severe toxic reactions resulting in fever, confusion, acutely lowered blood pressure, massive fluid retention in the lungs, and abnormal function of the liver and kidneys. Because newer approaches may reduce these effects, patients with therapy-resistant cancer are, nevertheless, encouraged to inquire about IL-2 therapy.

Tumor Necrosis Factor (TNF)

Another lymphokine (TNF) has some activity against tumors. The problems here are the same as with other immunotherapies, namely, benefits are unclear and severe toxic effects, such as extreme weight loss, are common. It is still uncertain when and how the drug should be used, but clinical trials are continuing. Recent experimental programs have combined TNF with standard chemotherapy to look for some beneficial effect.

Unproven Cures

In many cases, cancer cannot be cured by methods currently available. Patients are often faced with overwhelming odds. For example, they may have an 80 percent chance of death from their cancer and only 20 percent chance of cure or even long-term survival. When faced with these odds or when anticancer treatments have failed, some patients search for cures among unproven therapies.

Patients turn to these forms of treatment because they are desperate. They know that many common tumors are not curable by accepted therapy, and they think that all they have to look forward to is discomfort and ultimately death. Therefore, they feel they have nothing to lose. In this situation, patients will undergo irrational treatments that, in other circumstances, they would condemn as worthless. No reliable figures are available to show how much is spent on these quack cures, but it is probably several million dollars each year. About 5 percent of cancer patients seriously investigate or participate in these unproven therapies.

Treatments unrecognized by the medical profession and not approved by government agencies, such as the FDA, continue to offer unrealistic hope to cancer patients. Unproven therapies include diets to prevent or cure cancer, devices to treat cancer, unproven psychological management techniques, and unproven drugs or compounds. These quack drugs are not only unproven in human trials, but they are also unproven in animal tests or cell culture screens. In addition, there is no scientific or theoretical basis for their presumed activity against cancer. That is, they do not affect any biochemical process that might realistically kill tumor cells. Drugs in clinical trials for FDA approval have shown anticancer activity when they were tested in animals and cell cultures.

Unrecognized approaches all have one thing in common: they are ineffective against cancer. Diets or special foods will not cure cancer, nor will they prolong the survival of cancer patients. Devices referred to in this context are not approved by the FDA for use in therapy or surgery. Promoted as alternatives to standard forms of therapy, they appeal to terminal cancer patients who feel hopeless and frustrated that they have lost control over the disease and its treatment. Persons promoting diets and gadgets usually have a financial motive, and it is in their best interest to promise a successful outcome and tell the patient that he or she can influence the course of the disease.

The two most famous unproven cancer remedies of modern times were Krebiozen and Laetrile. Both drugs surfaced in the late 1940s and 1950s. Krebiozen is a substance claimed to have been isolated from beef blood. It was supposed to be a growth-controlling substance that killed or at least inhibited the growth of cancer cells. Thousands of patients, some of whom were receiving recognized chemotherapy, opted to take this substance since it seemed to offer the possibility of a cure. Investigations by the National Cancer Institute and the FDA eventually revealed that the substance being used was creatine, a common laboratory compound, and that it was useless in treating cancer. Use of the therapy gradually diminished when the public learned that it was worthless.

Laetrile is derived from apricot pits. Somehow this substance was supposed to be effective against cancer, and it was actually legalized for use in some states. Actually it is toxic, in part because under certain circumstances cyanide, a poison, is released when it is ingested. Nevertheless, thousands of patients used the drug and made the suppliers wealthy. Laboratory testing in animals and case reports of patients treated with the substance eventually revealed it to be useless. Outside the United States it is still being used despite its toxicity and lack of any benefit. The use of Laetrile bilked patients of their savings and prevented them from receiving accepted therapies that would have at least improved the quality of their lives.

Recently, an unproven type of immunotherapy has taken the place of Krebiozen and Laetrile. Promoters suggest that by modifying the immune system with a serum (plural, sera), a blood product sometimes produced with the aid of the patient's own tumor cells, a cancer cure or remission can be obtained. The appeal of this approach probably lies with its similarity to scientific research into the role of the immune system in protecting us from cancer. So far, legitimate research in this field has not produced any cures, and certainly there is no evidence that attempts to modify the immune system with sera or other compounds will cure cancer. The risk of contamination of sera with AIDS virus will prevent widespread use of these therapies. Apparently human sera from donors, which may be contaminated with AIDS virus, is combined with the patient's cells, perhaps to grow the cells in culture. In this way, the ultimate product made for injection may carry the AIDS virus. Most administrations of sera to cure cancer are done outside this country. However, some patients are desperate enough to travel to other countries, such as Mexico, where mysterious sera are injected with the mistaken hope of cures. The cost is usually in the thousands of dollars. Sometimes it is combined with standard chemotherapy, but legitimate immunotherapy as described earlier in this chapter should not be confused with the worthless quackery offered by promoters in mass media.

In the United States, control over drug therapies is strict. Sometimes this results in delay of approval for new anticancer drugs, but this is a small price to pay for safety and the assurance that the drug is beneficial. Other countries are more lax, so cancer treatment with unproven drugs, compounds, and sera continues. Patients cannot be too strongly discouraged from going outside the United States for this therapy. Besides the high risk of contamination and high cost of these treatments, there is no scientific evidence—such as properly controlled and analyzed clinical trials—that these unproven therapies can cure any patient of cancer.

The American Cancer Society and its hotlines, serviced by local chapters, and the National Cancer Institute (1-800-4-CANCER) maintain files of information about all unproven cancer treatments. They can answer any question concerning a proposed treatment and can inform you if the therapy is recognized by the medical profession. Once you know the facts about chemotherapy, you will most likely choose to undergo treatment with accepted therapies rather than seek out unproven treatments that promise more cures with less suffering.

If a cancer cure is found, your physician will know about it and the news media will broadcast its discovery almost instantaneously. In the meantime, unproven therapies can be potentially dangerous and very expensive.

Psychological Cures

Besides alternative chemotherapies and devices, psychological management techniques have been proposed as therapy for cancer patients. Relaxation, meditation, and other methods to improve mental outlook or encourage optimism are used by many cancer patients. It is inexpensive and without side effects, but it has never been shown in a properly run clinical trial that it cures cancer or even prolongs the life of cancer patients. Reasonable optimism can improve the quality of life. Many cancer centers promote support groups that may use some of these techniques to help patients cope or adapt to the diagnosis of cancer, or to improve the quality of life, but not to cure or treat their cancer. Counseling, group and individual psychotherapy, meditation, relaxation techniques, and self-help groups can support and benefit many patients. But legitimate uses of psychological techniques are sometimes perverted by individuals who claim that they will improve survival. When it is suggested, for example, that visualizing the tumor and imagining its destruction can actually shrink the cancer, that is a perversion of a legitimate relaxation technique. These unproven psychological management techniques can be harmful when they fail, because they make patients feel guilty about not trying hard enough. Patients are led to believe that if they had tried harder, their tumors would have diminished.

Mind-Body Relationships

Another questionable approach to cancer therapy depends on the effect of the mind on body functions, so-called mind-body relationships. Several popular books and many medical self-help magazines have suggested that these techniques can favorably affect the course of a patient's cancer. Research has yet to prove that influencing the mind can affect any part of the body, including the immune system, in a way that is ever likely to cure or significantly alleviate cancer. The same conclusion pertains to the relationship between stress and cancer. There is no scientific evidence that stress causes cancer, reactivates dormant cancer, or that relief of stress improves cancer prognosis.

Some evidence supports the beneficial effect of a positive attitude on the functioning of the immune system. A positive attitude means that the patient approaches therapy with the feeling that all will be well. A giant leap of faith is made, however, if a patient believes that such a positive attitude will allow the immune system to overcome and kill cancer cells. No such effect has ever been demonstrated, and it is unlikely that the mind will be found to exert a major influence on the immune system. There is nothing wrong, however, with hoping for a good outcome from chemotherapy and trying to be optimistic about the future.

CHAPTER 7

Dealing with Side Effects

Chapter 2 includes a summary of side effects for the most commonly used chemotherapy drugs. A quick look at this list shows that most of them have similar side effects. Common side effects are nausea, vomiting, and diarrhea, usually during the first day or two after chemotherapy is administered. This chapter describes chemotherapy side effects and how they can be treated, or prevented.

Control of Nausea and Vomiting

Mr. G., at age twenty-two, developed Hodgkin's disease, requiring treatment with adriamycin, bleomycin, vinblastine, and DTIC. Knowing that these drugs produce a great deal of vomiting, his nurse instructed him carefully about techniques (such as avoiding unpleasant smells or sudden movement) to prevent vomiting. One hour before therapy, Mr. G. took Trilafon orally and during his treatment received Trilafon

intravenously. Despite adequate oral and rectal doses of that
medication during the twenty-four hours after treatment,
severe vomiting occurred. On subsequent occasions,
intravenous dexamethasone and THC tablets also failed to
control his vomiting, so he began to miss appointments.
Finally, after a period of trial and error, he completed his
therapy with the aid of a complex program:

The night before his scheduled appointment, he took a
sedative and, on arising, a dose of Trilafon. Before his
chemotherapy, the nurse administered a barbiturate and
dexamethasone, and started an intravenous drip of Trilafon.
Because of the sedative effects of these drugs, he stayed
overnight in the hospital and received further doses of
Trilafon supplemented with intermittent doses of intravenous
Reglan. The next morning, he was able to resume his normal
activities and eventually completed his course of
chemotherapy.

Cancer patients fear uncontrolled nausea and vomiting from
chemotherapy almost as much as they do pain. They may even
decline potentially lifesaving chemotherapy because they anticipate
severe vomiting. For this reason, physicians and nurses are trained
to counsel patients from the beginning about techniques to avoid
these side effects. Also, they will use antiemetic (antivomiting) drugs
to control nausea and vomiting. Patients should understand that,
despite these precautions, some nausea or vomiting may occur, but
this side effect is a small sacrifice if the chemotherapy works. Based
on experience, the following measures, when carried out by patients
and their families, will prevent or at least control nausea and vomiting.

1. Do not fast before receiving chemotherapy. Fasting does nothing to prevent vomiting, and it interferes with good nutrition.
2. Avoid sights, sounds, smells, and images that could start a
vomiting reflex. For example, loud noises, strong smells, or messy
spills could trigger vomiting.

3. Avoid sudden changes in position, because this can cause motion sickness.

4. Avoid eating large meals during the period when nausea and vomiting are most likely to occur. Oncologists and oncology nurses can estimate the interval during which vomiting will occur. And after one or two cycles of chemotherapy, patients generally know when they are most likely to vomit. During this period, drink only small amounts of carbonated beverages, soups, or juices. Avoid liquids that are too hot or too cold. Use a straw to prevent unnecessary movement that could trigger vomiting. If you do vomit, wait several hours before taking more food or drink to prevent further retching.

5. Sleep. Vomiting rarely occurs while sleeping. Patients worry about breathing in vomited material, but this seldom happens unless they are extremely weak or overmedicated. Sleeping on one side reduces this risk.

6. Warn family and friends about the possibility of unexpected vomiting. Be prepared with basins, cleanup towels, and washable clothing and linens.

7. Practice relaxation techniques, especially if they have worked in the past for other medical or psychological problems. So-called mind-body or behavioral techniques, such as the relaxation response, biofeedback, or even hypnosis, have worked for patients. Relaxation techniques control the activity of the mind in order to control some functions of the body. The relaxation response is described by Dr. Herbert Benson in his book *The Relaxation Response*. The patient repeats a one-syllable word, trying to remain unaware of outside stimuli, without falling asleep. This results in a mind state during which minor to moderate degrees of nausea can be controlled, preventing vomiting.

Over time, some patients develop what is called anticipatory vomiting. They become queasy, nauseated, and even vomit as the time approaches for their next treatment. Such anticipatory vomiting often leads patients to refuse therapy and to miss appointments. To prevent this type of side effect, ask your doctor to give you a complete explanation of what to expect from therapy, a thorough review of ways to avoid nausea and vomiting, and a prescription for adequate antivomiting medications.

Patients almost always need medication to prevent nausea and vomiting. Phenothiazine drugs are generally used. These include Compazine (prochlorperazine), Torecan (thiethylperazine), and Trilafon (perphenazine). These drugs generally work by inhibiting the centers in the brain that control vomiting. Their main side effects are drowsiness and, much less frequently, abnormal involuntary movements of the head and neck. The head movements may be treated with antihistamines, which are sometimes given ahead of time to prevent this side effect. Most patients gain control of nausea by taking one dose orally one hour before treatment. Afterward, it is often sufficient to take one dose every three or four hours orally for nausea or rectally for vomiting. Dosing should continue until nausea has completely subsided. Too often patients do not take the posttreatment doses or stop taking the medication too soon, so they don't get full protection.

Chemotherapy does not cause the same degree of nausea and vomiting in all patients. Not all drugs cause nausea or vomiting. Some patients are unusually sensitive to chemotherapy, or they may be receiving severely toxic agents such as cisplatin, adriamycin, DTIC, nitrogen mustard, or actinomycin. Cortisonelike drugs, such as dexamethasone and methylprednisolone, may be given intravenously just before chemotherapy. Combined with phenothiazines, these drugs often help more sensitive patients avoid vomiting. The active ingredient in marijuana, THC, prevents vomiting in many younger patients. They find that inhalation of this drug or ingestion of THC tablets controls vomiting as well as or better than phenothiazines. However, psychological side effects, such as depersonalization, prevent widespread use. Truly resistant vomiting often responds well to large doses of Reglan (metoclopramide) administered orally or intravenously before treatment and then hours afterward; doctors sometimes combine Reglan with dexamethasone and phenothiazines for even greater control.

Besides the drugs mentioned, physicians have a long list of other agents to control vomiting, including tranquilizers (haloperidol, thorazine), sedatives (barbiturates, lorazepam), and Tigan (trimethobenzamide). Be assured that some combination of drugs will control this side effect.

Occasionally patients confuse vomiting from the cancer itself with that caused by chemotherapy. For example, a tumor that spreads to the brain or blocks the digestive tract can induce vomiting. Unusual vomiting or vomiting not preceded by nausea could mean that the disease, rather than the chemotherapy, may be the cause.

Diarrhea sometimes accompanies vomiting or occurs by itself. A light diet and use of Kaopectate, with or without paregoric, is all that is generally required to control this side effect. Contrary to popular belief, what a patient eats has little if any effect on his or her cancer. A light diet consists of clear soups, gelatin desserts, custards, baked potatoes, and noncitrus juices. Because vomiting caused by chemotherapy usually lasts only one to two days, it is not likely to affect the patient's nutrition. Occasionally, the drug Lomotil or Imodium is needed for diarrhea control. These drugs, however, can cause constipation if overused, or excessive cramping can result for no known reason. Patients must watch for dehydration, often manifested by a declining urine output.

Hair Loss

Hair loss is a frequent side effect caused by chemotherapy. The drugs most likely to cause hair loss include cyclophosphamide, vincristine, methotrexate, 5-fluorouracil (uncommon), adriamycin, daunomycin, and cisplatin. These drugs and some others destroy rapidly growing cancer cells, but they also affect other dividing cells, such as those in hair follicles. This causes hairs to break or fall out with even slight pulling or gentle brushing. Hair loss will be greater at higher doses or if the drugs are given in combination with each other.

Alopecia, the scientific term for hair loss, is perhaps the most emotionally distressing side effect of anticancer drug therapy. Hair is associated with sexual attractiveness, and hair loss is often equated with aging. Despite the potential emotional distress, however, most patients can cope with this side effect, particularly if they are properly informed as to when the loss will occur and how much hair loss to expect. Hair washing and brushing do not increase the amount of hair loss.

Usually the physicians and nurses treating a patient know the names and addresses of reputable wig makers who will design an affordable wig that looks natural. Wigs are tax deductible as medical expenses, and their cost is often covered, at least in part, by medical insurance. Sometimes reimbursement will be made if a physician writes a prescription for a wig. The American Cancer Society, hospitals, and other social service agencies will often help defray the expense if no reimbursement options exist. Most of all, remember that the loss is usually temporary and hair will eventually grow back.

There are three types of wigs: custom-made, customized, and ready-to-wear. Custom-made wigs are expensive, usually costing over $1,000 and possibly as much as $3,000. They are constructed from European hair, which is fine, as opposed to coarser Oriental hair. The foundation is made from lace and custom-fitted to the patient's scalp. Once fabricated, the wig is styled according to the patient's desires. Customized wigs are ready-made with good quality hair and are adjusted to hair style and head size. They will usually cost less than custom-made wigs. Ready-to-wear wigs are the least expensive, from $75 to $300. They come in many styles, colors, and materials. Nylon foundations used in these wigs may be hot in warm weather, and the hair is usually synthetic and coarse. It is sometimes difficult to get a good fit. Wigs are available for both men and women, but men are more likely to decline wearing one, since baldness is more socially acceptable in men than in women.

An often overlooked alternative to a wig is a turban. These head coverings can be attractive and fashionable. They are inexpensive, and some women purchase several, wearing varying styles and colors at different times.

Two methods are available to help minimize hair loss. In both methods, the object is to limit the amount of the chemotherapy drug that reaches the hair follicles. The first method involves using a modified blood pressure cuff, which is inflated around the patient's head at a pressure higher than the patient's blood pressure. A second way of restricting blood flow and, therefore, drug delivery to the hair follicles uses an ice pack to cover the entire scalp. Ice or chemical reactions supply the proper amount of cooling.

Both methods must be started a few minutes before infusing chemotherapy and maintained for ten to thirty minutes after the infusion is stopped. This limits the use of these methods to schedules in which the drugs are given over a relatively short period of time, certainly not when the drugs are administered over a twenty-four-hour period.

Hair loss prevention techniques vary widely among treatment centers. There are several reasons why some oncologists avoid these techniques unless specifically requested by their patients. First, there is worry in the case of leukemias, lymphomas, and certain solid tumors, such as breast cancer, that sanctuary areas will be created in the scalp where circulating cancer cells will be protected from exposure to the drug. These cells might then divide and form metastases in the scalp or other sites. Another consideration is patient comfort, particularly when drugs are infused over longer periods of time. Patients report pain and discomfort with prolonged scalp cooling, and it is theoretically possible to cause nerve damage if inflation pressures are too high. Finally, the effectiveness of these methods is questionable, since some patients report major hair loss despite such treatments.

Ask your physician about these methods if you are concerned about hair loss. Certainly, if infusion times are short, a trial of one or both of these methods is almost risk-free and can be stopped at any time if discomfort becomes severe. The risk of creating a sanctuary in the scalp or of causing nerve damage, although theoretically possible, is small.

There are a few simple measures you can take to care for remaining hair. These include cutting hair short to reduce pulling when combing or brushing, applying shampoo only once, washing less frequently, and avoiding permanents, coloring, and other hair treatments. There are no useful drugs available to prevent hair

loss, nor to speed regrowth. Minoxidil, recently approved by the
FDA for use in natural hair loss, has not yet been studied in patients
receiving cancer chemotherapy.

Mouth Care

One of the most distressing side effects of cancer chemotherapy is
mucositis, or inflammation of the mucous membranes of the mouth
and nearby areas, including the throat and esophagus. Patients
complain of severe mouth pain, foul taste, and lost sense of taste.
Ulcerations frequently occur after treatment with drugs that kill
rapidly multiplying cells, such as the cells that line the mucous
membranes. These painful ulcers may also occur after radiation
treatments and even in cancer patients who have not undergone
recent therapy, presumably as a result of a viral infection.

Severe mouth pain can occur in both treated and untreated cancer patients from any of a number of causes. For example, a thick
white covering on the tongue can be due to a yeastlike infection
with a fungus called *Candida albicans,* or thrush. A painful ulceration on the lip or the area adjacent to the lip, called a cold sore,
may represent infection with *Herpes simplex* virus. Tooth or gum
infections can also be very painful. Often, combinations of these
infections require treatment with a number of different drugs,
particularly if the exact cause is unknown.

An attempt should be made to prevent or reduce severe mouth
infections, because they are so debilitating and interfere with eating
and enjoyment of life. To prevent painful gum infections and tooth
pain, brush your teeth regularly with toothpaste or baking soda.
You should also maintain tooth fillings and correct any abscesses
or other dental abnormalities that could lead to infection. Continue
professional cleanings, use dental floss, and inspect your mouth
daily during and after chemotherapy treatments. Avoid foods that
are hot, spicy, acidic, or otherwise irritating, as well as alcohol,
tobacco, and commercial mouthwashes that tend to dry mucous
membranes. A diet high in protein, with adequate vitamins and
minerals, is essential to promote healing of the mucous membranes

of the mouth. Keep your mouth moist by drinking adequate fluids, sucking on sugarless hard candies, and chewing sugarless gum. Rinse with hydrogen peroxide to help maintain good mouth hygiene and preserve a feeling of cleanliness. Use hydrogen peroxide, either as a one-to-one dilution with water (one quarter cup of peroxide to one quarter cup of water) or as a mint-flavored preparation available over the counter in drugstores. Lipstick, lip balm, and petroleum jelly will keep the lips well moisturized.

Fungal infections of the tongue or throat due to *Candida albicans*—also known as yeast infections, thrush, or moniliasis—respond to lozenges or throat drops containing the antifungal agent clotrimazole (Mycelex Troche), or mouth rinses with a ready-made suspension of mycostatin (Nystatin), another antifungal drug. To prevent recurrences of *herpes simplex* infections, oral use of the antibiotic acyclovir (Zovirax) may be prescribed. This same antibiotic can be used intravenously to treat severe *herpes simplex* infections of the mouth and adjacent areas.

Once painful ulcers appear in the mouth, their cause can often be determined with a scraping of the mucous membranes taken with a wooden stick or a glass slide and then viewed under a microscope. Cultures for bacteria, fungi, and viruses help, but your physician should not wait for the results of these tests before starting to treat the infection. An antifungal drug, combined with hydrogen peroxide mouthwashes, is generally the first prescribed treatment.

Since most painful ulcers have no specific cause, painkillers applied directly to the sores can help, but they are usually not terribly effective and may cause gagging. The topical anesthetic Lidocaine, closely related to Novocain, is a thick, viscous solution that can be applied directly with a cotton-tipped applicator or diluted and used as a rinse. Unfortunately, the numbing effect is not tolerated by some patients, and they often gag when too much of the mouth and throat become numbed. Dyclone 1 percent and benzocaine are other anesthetic drugs that can be administered as a mouth rinse or as a spray from an atomizer. A solution of the antihistamine diphenhydramine (Benedryl) may also be used for its painkilling effect.

Many different drugs have been used to coat the sores, thereby preventing the pain caused by contact with saliva: antacids, milk of magnesia, Kaopectate, and Orabase. Orabase is a prescription medicine that coats the ulcer and resists removal by saliva. It is also available mixed with a corticosteroid (Kenalog), which prevents some of the inflammation that accompanies these ulcers. Recently, sucrafate (Carafate) has become available. This drug, commonly used to treat stomach ulcers, can be made into a solution by mashing the tablets in a small amount of water and then using the mixture as a mouth rinse. The drug sticks to ulcerated surfaces and prevents saliva from coming into contact with the ulcer. This mixture and antifungal agents can be swallowed to treat or prevent ulcerations farther down in the esophagus.

The most severe and painful ulcerations caused by chemotherapy often require three or four drugs of different types (antifungal, ulcer-coating, analgesic, and antiviral). Acyclovir, an anti–*herpes simplex* drug, is used more frequently, since many mouth ulcers prove by culture to be due to this virus. Narcotics, given orally or intravenously, are sometimes needed in severe, resistant cases. I cannot overemphasize the importance of preventive mouth care and dental hygiene, since diligent care can prevent much discomfort.

Nutrition

During chemotherapy, appetite declines and food may be the last thing the patient wants. Although adequate nutrition is important, sometimes family members make too much of it. They do this out of concern and because it is one of the few things that the patient and his or her loved ones can control.

Many books and pamphlets are available through the American Cancer Society with suggestions and recipes for good nutrition. During chemotherapy, it is necessary only to maintain weight or, at least, keep weight loss to a minimum and maintain adequate fluid intake. As long as the patient urinates a quart or more a day, it is unlikely that dehydration will become a problem.

Calories and vitamins lost can be made up during the rest periods built into the chemotherapy schedule. Supplemental feedings with either milk-based or milk-free products, such as the various formulations of Sustacal or Ensure, supply extra calories in a relatively concentrated form. Some patients tolerate milk-free supplements better than those that are milk-based. In contrast to these liquid supplements, Resource, another calorie supplement, comes as crystals to be dissolved in water before drinking. Patients need to try different brands and flavors before deciding whether these supplements are tolerable and helpful in maintaining weight. Appetite and enjoyment of food do return if chemotherapy is effective and the patient achieves partial or complete remission.

"Total parenteral nutrition" (TPN) means that all necessary nutrients are provided to the patient in liquids administered through intravenous infusion. Some patients show improved results when they receive TPN and chemotherapy at the same time. Generally, TPN has not been very helpful in improving survival statistics or quality of life. There are side effects and dangers as well, including infections and interference with normal metabolism. TPN is now administered primarily during first-line chemotherapy to patients who are unable to eat normally, such as those with head and neck cancers who have recently undergone surgery.

Anemia, Infection, and Bleeding

One group of chemotherapy drugs is called cytotoxic, because they interfere with cell metabolism, causing the cells to die. Certain normal cells in the human body are also very sensitive to these cytotoxic agents, for example, the cells of the mucous membranes in the mouth, cells lining the intestines, cells in the hair follicles, and cells in the bone marrow, located within the breastbone, ribs, spine, and skull. In general, therefore, the cytotoxic drugs usually cause a similar constellation of symptoms: mouth sores, diarrhea, hair loss, and bone marrow suppression.

Bone marrow cells normally develop into red blood cells, which carry oxygen; white blood cells, which defend the body against infection; and platelets, which prevent bleeding. Bone marrow suppression, therefore, can cause anemia, infection, or excessive bleeding.

Anemia

Suppression of the bone marrow causes lower red blood cell counts. Since red cells carry oxygen, reduction in the number of red cells results in decreased oxygen delivery to the body, a condition called anemia. If the anemia becomes severe, blood transfusions may be required to restore the number of red cells to normal levels.

Infection

Suppression of the bone marrow lowers white blood cell counts. White blood counts normally stay within an established range of values but, as chemotherapy proceeds, the white count may fall below this range. Once infection develops, the patient's temperature often goes up and the bone marrow normally produces more white blood cells to combat the infection. Patients with low white blood cell counts, therefore, have little natural resistance to infection.

When low white blood cell counts are expected, blood tests are taken to monitor the numbers. If they reach a dangerously low level likely to result in serious infection, the doses of chemotherapeutic drugs are reduced. Despite this precaution, many patients become infected. All the patient can do at this point is go to the hospital and receive intravenous antibiotics.

Even more important than the total white blood cell count is the number of white cells that are granulocytes, also called polys. A granulocyte count indicates the risk of acquiring an infection. The lower the granulocyte count, the greater the risk of infection. Most oncologists check the white blood cell count prior to giving chemotherapy.

After a period of one or more weeks of chemotherapy, the patient may lose the ability to produce white cells, resulting in lower resistance to infection. Fever, chills, sore throat, and cough are all symptoms of such infection. These symptoms must be reported promptly to the treating oncologist, so that laboratory testing can be done to identify the cause.

Blood cultures are usually taken to identify the bacteria or other organisms causing the infection. To do a blood culture, a sample of the patient's blood is drawn into a sterile container containing a special broth that allows the bacteria to grow and be identified. Cultures of urine, sputum, and other body fluids are also taken and examined. Another blood sample is taken at the same time so that blood cells can be counted. The blood cell count is generally available before the culture results. Therefore, if the white blood cell count is low, the physician cannot wait for the results of the cultures but must begin treatment, usually with broad-spectrum antibiotics. This means that one or more different antibiotics are given, usually by intravenous infusion, while the patient is in the hospital. Broad-spectrum antibiotics are effective against a wide range of organisms. Later, if an organism is isolated and identified, the antibiotics can be more exactly tailored to destroy that particular organism.

Many infections can be life-threatening because the bacteria may actually enter the blood. Learn to recognize the early symptoms, and inform your oncologist if they occur. If there's any temperature elevation, waiting too long can be fatal. Some of the more common symptoms of serious infection are: fever greater than 100.5°F (38.3 °C); shaking chills; sweating at night; severe diarrhea; and sore throat. If infection is suspected, intravenous antibiotics, often more than one, are administered until an alternative reason for the symptoms is known or the infection is eliminated.

There is little the patient can do, while his or her white count is low, to prevent infection. It helps to avoid crowds and family members or friends who are sick. Frequent hand washing is effective because many viruses and bacteria are spread by touching contaminated hands, followed by hand-to-nose contact. Many times, the infection is caused by bacteria normally residing in the patient's intestines. The anal region is a common site for infections. Gentle wiping and the use of moistened cleansing tissues may help reduce the potential for infection in this area. A bidet, if available, can help maintain cleanliness of the anal and genital areas.

Antibiotics taken orally may help prevent infections in some patients with leukemia, but most patients receiving chemotherapy do not take antibiotics. The oncologist will decide in individual cases whether to prescribe antibiotics on a preventive basis. Some are expensive, and others may not work to prevent infection. One risk of antibiotic therapy is that the organism causing the infection will become resistant to the antibiotic used and to other antibiotics as well, making it difficult to treat.

Patients whose bone marrow has been or will be severely suppressed by chemotherapy may stay in specially constructed rooms that are kept relatively free of bacteria. It is not entirely clear whether this limited ability to prevent infection is worth the high cost. Leukemia patients and those undergoing bone marrow transplantation often use such rooms.

Bleeding

Bone marrow suppression also decreases the patient's platelet count. Platelets are cells, produced like red cells and white cells in the bone marrow, about which researchers know very little. Their primary function is to prevent excessive bleeding.

Because chemotherapy suppresses the marrow, fewer platelets are produced. Reduction to a level below 20,000 per cubic millimeter can result in bleeding from the gums, nose, skin, intestines, or other locations. Bleeding must be treated immediately with platelets obtained from normal blood donors.

Low platelet counts can result in serious bleeding into various organs of the body. If the bleeding is in the intestines, stools can become red or black and tarlike. If the bleeding is in the kidneys or urinary tract, the urine will become red. If it is in the brain, headache, paralysis, and unconsciousness may result. Bleeding can show itself almost anywhere. Sometimes serious bleeding is heralded by nosebleeds, bleeding gums, red spots on the skin or inside the mouth, or black-and-blue marks on the skin. Ask your oncologist what signs and symptoms indicate significant bleeding. In general, however, any evidence of bleeding should be reported to your physician immediately.

Certain over-the-counter drugs interfere with platelet function and may increase the potential for bleeding, particularly when platelet counts are low. These drugs include: aspirin, aspirin-containing medicines, Alka-Seltzer, for example; Ibuprofen, marketed under trade names such as Medipren, Advil, or Nuprin; antihistamines; and the cough medicine Robitussin. Once bleeding has started, the patient must be hospitalized to receive transfusions to make up for his or her loss of red cells and platelets.

You can reduce the incidence of bleeding by using special care when shaving and brushing your teeth, by avoiding heavy-duty gardening or contact sports, and by preventing burns while ironing or cooking. A serious nosebleed may be prevented by blowing your nose gently, without pressing on the nostrils, and by keeping the lining of the nose moist with a vaporizer or glycerin gently applied with a cotton swab.

Anaphylaxis

Occasionally, patients will have acute drug reactions at the time chemotherapy is administered. These so-called anaphylactic reactions cause wheezing and breathing difficulty. Blood pressure drops suddenly, leading to shock and even death if not treated immediately. In special oncology units, drugs and equipment are available to treat these severe and potentially fatal drug reactions. If a drug is known to cause this type of reaction, doctors administer only small test doses, with emergency equipment standing by, before attempting to give full doses.

Lung Problems

Some patients have lung difficulties with chemotherapy drugs. Usually the first symptoms are wheezing or shortness of breath. Chest X rays and special lung function testing are used to diagnose the problem and, if necessary, the drug will be discontinued. Your physician may prescribe medications to treat wheezing and shortness of breath if these symptoms appear immediately after chemotherapy is administered. Medications are also available to prevent this complication if it seems likely to happen again or for long-term treatment if the symptoms persist. Ask your physician about these medications. Rarely, permanent lung damage resulting in difficulty breathing can occur as a serious side effect.

Kidney and Liver Problems

Many chemotherapy drugs cause kidney and liver problems. To prevent kidney dysfunction, the patient should drink large amounts of fluids before and after treatment. With some drugs, extra fluids are given intravenously just prior to administration of chemotherapy. Leg swelling, a symptom of fluid retention caused by inadequate kidney function, should be reported promptly. Liver problems are indicated by yellowing of the skin and eyes—a condition called jaundice—and dark urine. Unfortunately, there is no known way to prevent these liver complications.

Neurological (Nervous System) Problems

Neurological (nervous system) problems may also occur. Symptoms include sharp shooting pains in the arms, legs, or both; tingling in fingers or toes; constipation; or difficulty walking. It is important to report any such problem, since it could be a side effect of chemotherapy. The only treatment for these symptoms is to discontinue the drug. Rarely, a patient's nervous system may be seriously injured, resulting in paralysis or loss of an important function, such as hearing or balance. In this instance, physical and occupational therapy may help, but serious nerve damage is likely to be irreversible.

Skin Rashes

A few patients develop skin rashes and skin darkening in response to chemotherapy. Not much is known about why these abnormalities develop, and, unfortunately, not much can be done about them, except to stop the drug if symptoms become severe.

A few drugs (adriamycin, for example) cause radiation recall. In these instances, skin areas that have been previously exposed to radiation become inflamed and even ulcerated a short time after chemotherapy is started. The condition is painful but usually not serious. Occasionally skin grafting is required, but the condition generally heals after the drug is discontinued.

Second Malignancies

Finally, some drugs can cause second malignancies, usually years after the patient completes treatment. Second malignancies commonly occur as leukemia, lymphoma, or sarcoma. They can be treated with chemotherapy, but their cure rate is low. Although little can be done to prevent this complication, patients should ask about the risk. Almost always, however, the expected benefit of therapy will outweigh the risk of a second malignancy. There are several reasons for this: (1) second malignancies are not common, occurring in only 5 to 10 percent of patients receiving chemotherapy, usually after seven to ten years; (2) it is important to try to cure the patient, and certainly you cannot worry about a second malignancy if the patient does not survive the first; and (3) there is usually a period of three or more years before the risk of a second malignancy is significant, and many patients may not live that long, despite the use of chemotherapy.

Infertility

Some chemotherapy drugs affect fertility. Particular treatments call for drugs that also kill cells in the ovaries or testicles and cause sterility.

If a patient is pregnant, certain drugs present a special risk to the fetus, especially in early pregnancy. Some drugs cause miscarriages or birth defects. Often, a pregnant patient must consider undergoing an abortion before chemotherapy can begin. Before giving chemotherapy to women of child-bearing age, therefore, it is standard practice to do a pregnancy test. Fortunately, young women of child-bearing age do not often get cancer. Nevertheless, if a patient knows or suspects that she is pregnant, it is crucial that she tell her physician or oncologist.

Many of the drugs used to treat cancer cause infertility in men and women by destroying sperm-producing cells in the testes and eggs in the ovaries. The likelihood of causing infertility depends on the drugs used, the age of the patient, the number of drugs used, and the total doses administered. Using chemotherapy combined with radiation to reproductive organs probably increases the incidence of infertility. Infertility caused by chemotherapy cannot be prevented; therefore, patients wishing to have children and who require therapy with drugs known to cause infertility must bank their eggs or sperm for later use. They may then participate in artificial means of becoming pregnant, such as artificial insemination. These procedures may or may not be acceptable to some religious faiths, so patients often consult with their religious adviser before deciding to store sperm or eggs.

At present, egg preservation is possible only in research facilities. Unfertilized eggs store poorly and are difficult to fertilize successfully so that a normal pregnancy results later on. More research and experience is needed before egg storage can be recommended as an option for cancer patients.

Sperm banking is available in most large cities but is expensive, and it may be necessary to travel to a reliable facility. Before banking, a laboratory analysis is done to determine the number and activity level of the patient's sperm to ensure that useful quantities will be available for later use. Often cancer patients, those with Hodgkin's disease or testicular cancer, for example, have low sperm counts and abnormalities in the appearance of their sperm. They may be infertile as a result of their cancer. The sperm specimens are stored at very low temperatures in liquid nitrogen. Thawed sperm is artificially inseminated into the patient's female partner after cancer therapy has been completed. Not all inseminations produce pregnancies, even if sufficient numbers of sperm have been preserved.

Anticancer drugs also increase the likelihood of birth defects, particularly when given early in pregnancy. For this reason also, many pregnant cancer patients choose to have abortions before starting chemotherapy. Here, again, patients may wish to consult with their religious advisers concerning the issues involved in a therapeutic abortion. The patient's desires and the risks of continuing the pregnancy must be carefully considered and discussed fully with the oncologist before any action is taken.

The drugs most commonly associated with infertility are nitrogen mustard, cyclophosphamide, chlorambucil, busulfan, methotrexate, procarbazine, vincristine, and vinblastine. A number of factors affect the level of risk. Patients over thirty are more likely to become infertile than younger patients. The risk of infertility is greater if multiple drugs are used or if the patient receives radiotherapy to the reproductive organs along with chemotherapy. Infertility is more likely when larger cumulative doses of drug are used. It has been observed that patients with Hodgkin's disease and possibly other cancers are often infertile for no known reason before starting therapy.

Fertility issues are most important to younger patients who have not started families. Generally they accept chemotherapy if it is likely to help their illness and take measures to enable them to have children later on. Men may bank their sperm. Women with Hodgkin's disease can have their ovaries surgically moved out of radiation fields, or they can take birth control pills during radiotherapy. Hormones in birth control pills somehow protect the reproductive organs, decreasing the possibility of permanent infertility. Unfortunately surgery and hormones do not always work, and not much else can be done at the present time to prevent chemotherapy or radiotherapy from causing infertility.

It may be necessary to remove reproductive organs, such as in a hysterectomy or removal of the testes. Radiation can cause reproductive organs to fail, as when radiotherapy is delivered to the ovaries or testicles. To date, these radiotherapy patients are not considered candidates for the most modern infertility treatments, but this may change in the future.

Sexual Problems

Traditional sexual functioning is, obviously, impaired by removing primary sexual organs, such as the vagina or testes. Sexual activity or interest may also be affected if a patient's body is altered by surgery or radiation. For example, removal or irradiation of a breast may make a woman feel she is less desirable. The presence of various surgical devices can interfere with sexual activity. For example, some patients require an external colostomy, in which the end of the colon is made to exit the body through the abdomen, allowing intestinal waste to empty into a bag. Narcotics used for pain control may cause impotence.

How much dysfunction will occur and how likely the patient will adjust to the situation depends on many factors. It appears that previous sexual functioning is a predictor of adjustment to these types of treatment. Patients with active sex lives prior to cancer treatment are very inventive and often find ways to continue their mutually satisfying sex lives. Intercourse may give way to other pleasurable activities, such as caressing, kissing, or manual stimulation.

Emotional problems can prevent patients from resuming sexual activities they enjoyed before learning that they have cancer. They may have pain, fatigue, or shortness of breath because of lung surgery. They may be refocusing emotional energies on bodily sensations or changes, or on the need to prepare for death. Pain, if present, is difficult to ignore, and painkillers may cause fatigue and sleepiness. Sexual pleasure can distract from mild pain, but not from more significant discomfort.

Some physical abnormalities and symptoms can be treated. Decreased vaginal lubrication following radiation to this area can be helped with lubricants, such as K-Y Jelly. Breast implants are available that feel and look much like real breasts. Implantable penile prostheses aid men left impotent by prostatic surgery or radiation therapy. Before sexual activities are abandoned, patients should discuss the matter with a physician or sex therapist.

All too often, the problems are emotional rather than physical. The patient feels that his or her body has been mutilated or made unattractive. Sexual problems previously present in the relationship become magnified with the stresses of a cancer diagnosis and the rigors of its treatment. Counseling can help, but it is often difficult, with all else that is occurring, to find time for such therapy. Patients with no hope of recovery may be so depressed and anxious that they are incapable of emotionally demanding functions such as sex. To them, coping with death and dying takes priority over resuming a normal sex life. Families of these patients may find it extremely difficult to maintain an affectionate, loving relationship under these trying circumstances.

CHAPTER 8

Special Procedures

Venous Access Devices

Intravenous chemotherapy requires infusion of the drug into a vein. In other words, it requires venous access. Intravenous chemotherapy usually causes scars to develop on a patient's veins, making it progressively more difficult to administer treatments. This effect is also common in elderly patients and patients whose lymphatic systems have been damaged by tumor, surgery, or radiation. Sometimes the drugs themselves cause painful inflammation of veins, making them unusable. The current trend toward infusing chemotherapy over a longer period of time is another factor that makes it more difficult to maintain venous access.

For these reasons, two methods of administering chemotherapy with a catheter or tube that remains in a vein for weeks or months have been developed. These devices can be repeatedly punctured without scarring or collapsing the veins. They deliver drugs into large veins that are less likely than smaller veins to become inflamed or to collapse. Such devices dramatically improve the quality of life, since needle punctures to obtain blood or give chemotherapy are drastically curtailed.

One of the first of these indwelling catheters is the Hickman line. It is a flexible, hollow tube that is inserted through the skin of the chest, tunneled under the skin—to avoid infection—and then threaded through a large vein into the right atrium, or first chamber, of the heart. The other end of the catheter is coiled and stored in a pouch attached to the skin. Catheters of various sizes are currently available. Some have two central passages to allow two fluids to pass through simultaneously. Blood products, chemotherapy drugs, antibiotics, nutrients, and other fluids can be infused into these lines, and blood can be easily withdrawn for testing.

There are potential complications in relation to the use of indwelling catheters. The most feared is infection inside the catheter or at its tip. If this is suspected, it is necessary either to start aggressive antibiotic therapy or to remove the catheter. If one of the passages becomes obstructed by a blood clot, an enzyme called streptokinase is used to destroy the clot. To prevent such problems dressings must be changed daily, and the catheter must be flushed with heparin, an anticoagulant, to keep the line open and free of blood clots.

The second type of venous access device is the totally implantable indwelling venous catheter. These devices require less maintenance and, therefore, cost less than Hickman lines. The Port-a-Cath is one example; other equally satisfactory types are also available. Totally implantable devices consist of two parts. The first is a catheter that is threaded under the skin into a large vein and then into the atrium of the heart, as with the Hickman line. But instead of the other end exiting through the skin, it is attached to a second part, a reservoir, or port, placed under the skin in a surgically produced pouch. The port is a small container made of metal or plastic, covered by a self-sealing silicone membrane. A special needle is introduced through the skin and then through the membrane until the tip hits the solid wall of the container. Once secured in this position, fluids and blood products can be infused without repeatedly sticking needles into the patient's veins. Clotting can occur with this device as well, but usually only after hundreds of needle sticks.

The same complications—infection and clotting—occur as with the Hickman line. Cosmetically, however, it looks better and, since the catheter does not protrude outside the skin, it requires less maintenance than a Hickman line. Daily flushing with heparin, for example, is not necessary with this device. One disadvantage to the totally implantable device is the pain of the needle passing through the skin. If frequent venous access or continuous infusion therapy is required, the needle can be secured in place so that daily punctures are not necessary. As with the Hickman line, blood samples can be withdrawn for test purposes through these devices. The cost of either type of venous access device is usually covered by insurance.

High-Dose Methotrexate with Leucovorin Rescue

Methotrexate is a commonly used chemotherapy drug. It can be administered orally or intravenously. Methotrexate destroys cancer cells, but it can also be severely toxic to normal cells, such as those in mucous membranes or bone marrow. With most chemotherapy, side effects can usually be managed. With methotrexate, however, the patient may die from the drug's toxic effects.

Methotrexate's anticancer effects and its side effects depend on several factors.

• *The dose.* The patient will not die if the drug is given, intravenously or orally, at the usual doses. If large doses are given, however, irreversible changes occur in the bone marrow, mucous membranes, and gastrointestinal tract, ultimately causing death by infection, bleeding, or severe metabolic imbalances.

• *How often it is given.* If the patient receives the drug repeatedly over a prolonged period of time, irreversible and fatal liver damage may result. This can occur even when each individual dose is relatively small.

- *How it is administered.* The drug is more toxic if it is given orally than if it is given intravenously. Therefore, a dose easily tolerated by intravenous injection can be fatal if administered orally. For this reason, methotrexate is usually administered intravenously.

Methotrexate is removed from the body by the kidneys, and it is important for the kidneys to rid the body of the methotrexate before it can cause severe side effects. In the process, the drug can damage the kidneys, preventing this excretion. The chances of kidney damage are greater if the methotrexate level in the blood is high. So a vicious cycle begins as the methotrexate injures the kidneys, the kidneys excrete less methotrexate, blood levels of methotrexate get higher, the kidneys are further damaged by the high levels, and so on. For this reason, blood tests must be done to monitor kidney function whenever high doses of methotrexate are administered. If the situation is not corrected, the patient will die of kidney failure and from the other toxic effects of methotrexate. The presence of fluid collections in lung or abdomen precludes the use of high-dose methotrexate.

Small doses of methotrexate can be given without any special precautions; moderate and large doses require use of an antidote, leucovorin (also called citrovorum factor or folinic acid). Leucovorin is given twenty-four hours after the methotrexate infusion to shield, or rescue, normal cells from toxic effects of the drug. The leucovorin is given orally unless the patient is vomiting, when it is given intravenously.

Acute lymphocytic leukemia, osteogenic sarcoma, breast cancer, non-Hodgkin's lymphoma, and head and neck cancer may be treated with methotrexate. High-dose methotrexate therapy is controversial, and some oncologists believe that it probably has no therapeutic advantages over standard doses of the drug. If given, however, large doses of methotrexate also require leucovorin rescue. In addition, the urine must be made alkaline—that is, it must have pH value over 7—to help the kidneys excrete the methotrexate. To alkalinize the urine, the patient takes baking soda tablets—sodium bicarbonate—and then frequently tests his or her urine alkalinity, using dipsticks provided for that purpose. Intravenous leucovorin rescue is done at twenty-four hours after starting methotrexate infusion, followed by oral doses every six hours. Kidney function and blood levels of methotrexate are closely monitored. If kidney function deteriorates or if methotrexate levels do not fall as expected, it may be necessary to continue treatment with leucovorin at higher doses and for a longer period of time, even for fourteen days. Toxicity can also be reduced by increasing fluid intake, either orally or intravenously, before and after methotrexate treatment.

Patients receiving methotrexate must get written instructions and emergency numbers to call for advice. They need to know how to time their rescue tablets, how to use their alkalinization tablets, when to return for follow-up visits and blood tests, and what to do if side effects occur. Patients must be punctilious about taking the rescue medication on time and report any sign of toxicity (vomiting, diarrhea, or mouth sores). If such signs appear, the patient must report immediately to the treatment facility for blood tests to measure kidney function (serum creatinine) and methotrexate level.

Radiation Therapy

Many types of radiation can be used to treat cancer. Modern machines generate radiation energy suitable for treating different tumors at varying depths within the body. You do not need to know the physics involved in delivering radiation to cancers, but you should be aware of what radiation therapy can do and that it can be combined with drugs to destroy some tumors. Radiation therapy is useful when the tumor is known to be sensitive to the effects of radiation and when the disease is localized to a relatively small area. As the amount of tissue to be treated increases, side effects also increase. Treating more than one area is also difficult and usually results in toxicity, either immediately or sometime after treatment.

Many cancers are treated by a combination of chemotherapy with radiotherapy. Because side effects of both are similar, the risks of developing nausea, vomiting, anemia, infection, bleeding, or other symptoms are greater whenever radiation is used immediately before, immediately after, or during chemotherapy. Only experienced oncologists should supervise the delivery of such combination therapy.

The radiation is produced by large machines that allow the patient to be exposed for a short time to an intense beam of energy. This beam can penetrate deep into the body or it can be modified to treat lesions on or just beneath the skin. The patient lies on a table while the energy is delivered to the target area. There is no pain and the treatment lasts for only minutes. The skin may burn and flake off or show some change in color, but, if properly applied, radiation should not cause the skin to become scarred.

Patients should be asked to consider radiation alone, as an alternative to chemotherapy, when they have bone pain from metastases; blocked outflow tracts from the liver, gallbladder, kidney, or lymph nodes; or when large veins or arteries are obstructed. Painful tumors located near the body's surface or inside the body often disappear, at least temporarily, with radiation treatment.

The major potential advantages of radiation therapy over chemotherapy include: (1) there are fewer side effects if the tissue area treated is not too large; (2) only four to six weeks of treatment are usually required, whereas chemotherapy may take months (although, of course, chemotherapy treats more disease sites); and (3) if the tumor is sensitive to radiation, the response is often relatively long-lasting.

Transfusion Therapy

During chemotherapy, it is often necessary to transfuse blood products, such as red blood cells or platelets, obtained from blood donors. Some malignancies cause anemia, which, in turn, makes patients feel fatigued and unable to carry on their normal tasks. This is particularly true of blood and lymph node diseases, such as leukemia and lymphoma, but also occurs in the late stage of almost any cancer. Transfusing red blood cells can correct anemia.

Similarly, in some cancer patients, transfusing platelets helps to control bleeding and prevent strokes due to bleeding in the brain.

Initially patients do not like the idea of receiving transfusions. They fear AIDS, hepatitis, and other infectious diseases potentially transmitted by blood transfusions. These risks are small, however, with the use of volunteer donors and screening of blood products for evidence of AIDS and other viral infections, like hepatitis B.

The procedure for receiving a transfusion is simple. First, a blood sample is obtained from the patient for use in matching the patient's blood type with that of the donated blood. This may take several hours, so some patients leave a sample and return the next day for the actual transfusion. The blood product, usually in a bag, is hung at the bedside and a tubing line from the bag is attached to either an indwelling venous access device or to a needle that is then inserted into a vein in the patient's arm or hand. It usually takes about two to three hours to transfuse one bag of blood product. Following transfusion, or even during it, the patient may develop fever or hives. Acetaminophen for the fever and antihistamine for the hives generally take care of these side effects. More severe reactions should be reported immediately to the treating oncologist.

Transfusion therapy alone, as an alternative to chemotherapy, is considered for elderly patients, who cannot tolerate treatment of acute leukemia or other cancer, but who can be functional if their red blood cell count is maintained with red cell transfusions and their bleeding is prevented with platelet transfusions.

Bone Marrow Transplantation

Bone marrow is a tissue located inside certain bones—ribs, spine, skull, breastbone, and hips—where blood cells are made. These cells include red cells that carry oxygen to the body, white cells that defend the body against infection, and platelets that prevent excessive bleeding. If bone marrow is damaged, or suppressed, usually by high-dose radiation or chemicals, the marrow stops producing blood cells and life-threatening symptoms—anemia, overwhelming infection, and severe bleeding—can occur. Bone marrow transplantation (BMT) is a new procedure, developed in the 1970s, that is intended to replace damaged bone marrow with functioning bone marrow.

A patient receiving chemotherapy may receive large doses of toxic drugs to cure the cancer. Bone marrow transplantation is used to rescue the patient from the life-threatening toxic effects that such therapy can have. For example, a patient with acute leukemia receives large doses of busulfan or cyclophosphamide, combined with potentially fatal doses of radiotherapy, in an attempt to destroy the cancer. This therapy may well destroy most, if not all, of the leukemia cells, but it also completely destroys the patient's normal marrow cells. To prevent the patient from dying, bone marrow transplantation is done. Marrow may be donated by a genetically matched sibling or, if the patient has been put into complete remission with prior chemotherapy (by using a program described in Chapter 5), the patient's own marrow can be used.

Patients with leukemia, lymphoma, and breast cancer are currently the best candidates for bone marrow transplantation. It is very expensive, often costing $75,000 or more, and not all insurance companies cover the costs of the procedure, because they feel it is experimental and no more effective than standard chemotherapy. The cure rates are changing so rapidly that reliable figures cannot be given here but are available from your oncologist. He or she will suggest which high-dose chemotherapy program and which type of bone marrow transplantation might be best for you.

Autologous Marrow Transplantation (AMT)

If the patient's own marrow is used, the procedure is called autologous marrow transplantation (AMT). The marrow is removed from the patient after remission is obtained, but before he or she receives high doses of drugs or radiation. These doses are calculated to destroy all tumor cells. However, the doses are high enough to be potentially fatal unless the marrow is reinfused into the patient when the chemotherapy and radiotherapy end.

In some instances, it may be necessary to remove any malignant cells that may be present in the marrow from the cancer being treated. After removal from the patient, the marrow is treated with chemicals or with monoclonal antibodies, biologically prepared substances directed against antigens on the malignant cells. The cleaned-up marrow is stored and returned to the patient later to restore marrow functioning. Bone marrow cleanup is an experimental procedure that shows promise for increasing the usefulness of bone marrow transplants in cancer, especially lymphomas.

The advantage of AMT is that there is no need to find a genetically matched donor. The disadvantage is that living cancer cells may be reinfused into the patient, despite attempted cleanup procedures.

Genetically Matched Marrow Transplantation

If the marrow is taken from someone else and then given to the patient, the donor must be genetically matched. The best match is an identical twin, the next best is a brother or sister, and after that an unrelated person. Genetic matching is done by testing blood samples from the donor and the patient. A bone marrow registry is kept by blood bank networks throughout the United States to help locate compatible donors.

The advantage of taking marrow from a genetically matched donor is that no cancer cells are present in the infused marrow. The disadvantage is that the donor cells may react against the patient's cells, such as those in the skin or lining of the gastrointestinal tract, causing severe rashes and diarrhea.

Bone Marrow Transplantation Procedures

Regardless of the source of the marrow, the procedures for taking marrow out, storing it, thawing it, and giving it back to the patient are the same. The marrow is obtained from the donor or patient under general anesthesia, since the procedure involves drawing marrow out into syringes through needles inserted into multiple sites in the pelvic bones. There is little risk, except for the very rare reaction to anesthesia. The sites of marrow removal will be sore for about twenty-four to forty-eight hours.

The marrow consists of cells suspended in a liquid. It is placed into vials and stored frozen in liquid nitrogen. When the time comes to infuse it into the patient, the marrow is thawed by warming the vials. The marrow is transferred into a syringe or plastic bag, an intravenous tube is connected, and the marrow is infused by gravity into the patient's vein.

The marrow cells travel through the patient's blood, finding their way into the marrow cavities. Unfortunately, it takes three to four weeks for the reinfused marrow to grow and fill the marrow cavities with normal cells. During this period, patients may suffer painful infections and bleeding. The patient needs platelet transfusions during this so-called aplastic phase until new platelets are made from the infused bone marrow. Antibiotics are almost always needed to treat infections in these patients until new white blood cells develop from the transplanted marrow.

Appendix A

Informed Consent Form

(Fictitious and abbreviated example.)

Protocol number: 87-098
Protocol name: Breast Adjuvant Therapy
Patient's name: _____
Hospital number: _____

1. Rationale
   You have elected to receive radiation and chemotherapy for breast cancer. The purpose of this study is to determine whether chemotherapy should be given before or after radiation to the breast. Presently it is not known what sequence of therapy is most beneficial to patients like yourself. Half the patients in this study will receive radiation followed by chemotherapy; the other half will receive chemotherapy followed by radiotherapy.
   (More explanation would follow.)

2. Descriptions of Treatment to Be Undertaken
   If you are assigned to receive chemotherapy, it will be given two

weeks after completion of radiotherapy. The chemotherapy will consist of four drugs. The drugs will be given on an outpatient basis. There will be six three-week cycles. You will be followed with physical examinations, blood work, X rays, and nuclear medicine scans. No further treatment for your breast cancer will be necessary unless the disease recurs.

(More explanation, particularly of planned radiotherapy, would follow.)

3. Expected Benefits of Treatment

The expected benefit of the radiation treatment is eradication of the tumor while preserving a satisfactory appearance of the breast. The chemotherapy is expected to prevent recurrence of the tumor, or at least delay its reappearance.

(More explanation of benefits would follow.)

4. Side Effects and Risks

General side effects: You can anticipate loss of some or all of your hair. Nausea and vomiting are likely to occur after each treatment. The effect on your bone marrow will make you susceptible to infections and bleeding.

(More general side effects would be explained.)

In this study you will receive four drugs. Each has its own side effects:

A. Cyclophosphamide—This drug can cause irritation of the bladder and blood in the urine. Drinking large amounts of fluids before and after treatment will help prevent this side effect.

(More side effects discussed.)

B. Adriamycin—This drug can cause _____

C. Methotrexate—This drug can cause _____

D. 5-Fluorouracil—This drug can cause _____

(Side effects and measures to minimize them would follow for each drug.)

5. Alternatives

Alternative therapy that could be considered given the nature of your disease includes:

A. Further surgery (modified radical mastectomy) instead of radiation.

B. Surgery without follow-up radiation or chemotherapy. This would eliminate the possibility of preventing or delaying recurrence with chemotherapy.

(Other alternatives would be listed.)

Confidential information contained in your record will not be released without your consent.

(Other confidentiality issues would be outlined here.)

This hospital has no formal program for compensating patients or providing treatment for unanticipated medical injury arising from this research.

(Any informal programs might be listed here.)

At any point in this program, if there are any questions about your treatment, rights, risks, benefits, or alternative procedures, a representative of the Human Rights Protection Committee is available to speak with you (234-0000).

(Any other issues would be addressed here.)

I have fully explained to the Patient, _____, the nature and purpose of the treatment program described above and its risks.

_____   _____
Date   Physician's Name

I have been fully informed about the procedures to be followed, including alternative treatments, potential benefits, possible discomforts, and risks. In signing this consent form I agree to this method of treatment, and I understand that I am free to withdraw at any time and have this treatment discontinued, without prejudice of any kind. I also understand that if I have any questions at any time, they will be answered.

I have been given a copy of this consent form.

_____   _____
Witness   Signature of Patient

Appendix B

Cancer Service Agencies

American Cancer Society, Inc.
1599 Clifton Road
Atlanta, GA 30329
1-800-952-7430
1-404-320-3333
Services, support, referrals, rehabilitation, transportation.

Camps for children with cancer
Contact local or regional American Cancer Society office
List of camps for children who have or have had cancer.

Cancer Information Service
Office of Cancer Communications
National Cancer Institute
Bethesda, MD 20205
1-800-4-CANCER
Hawaii: 524-1234
Washington, D.C.: 636-5700
New York City: 794-7982
Alaska: 1-800-638-6070
Information, referral.

CanSurmount
Contact local American Cancer Society office
Group support, education.

I Can Cope
Contact local American Cancer Society office
Education, group support.

International Association of Laryngectomes
Contact local American Cancer Society office
Support groups, information. Concerned primarily with patients who have had laryngectomies.

Leukemia Society of America, Inc.
733 Third Avenue
New York, NY 10017
1-800-284-4271
1-212-573-8484
Information, support groups, referrals, transportation. Concerned primarily with leukemia patients and those suffering from related malignancies of blood and lymph nodes.

Make Today Count
P.O. Box 303
Burlington, IA 52601
1-319-753-6521
Support groups.

National Coalition for Cancer Survivorship
323 Eighth Street SW
Albuquerque, NM 87102
1-505-764-9956

Information, resources, political action and excellent newsletter including lists of resources.

National Hospice Organization
Suite 901
1901 North Moore Street
Arlington, VA 22209
1-800-658-8898
1-703-243-5900
National clearinghouse for locating hospice programs and information about hospice care.

Reach to Recovery
Contact local American Cancer Society office
Support group for breast cancer patients.

Support groups
Contact local or regional American Cancer Society office
Support groups are continually being formed to aid patients with cancer and to aid patients with specific cancers. Adult and children's groups. Meeting places and phone numbers often change.

United Ostomy Association, Inc.
2001 West Beverly Boulevard

Los Angeles, CA 90057
1-213-413-5510
*Information, support groups,
concerned primarily with patients having colostomies, il-
iostomies, or similar
operations.*

**Wish fulfillment organiza-
tions**
Contact local or regional
American Cancer Society
office
*Grants wishes for critically or
terminally ill children. List of
organizations serving local
area is usually available.*

Appendix C

Cancer Treatment Centers

National

National Cancer Institute
National Institutes of
  Health
Bethesda, MD 20892

Alabama

University of Alabama Medical Center
Comprehensive Cancer Cen-
  ter
619 South Nineteenth
  Street
Birmingham, AL 35233

Arizona

University of Arizona Health
  Services Center Cancer
  Center
1501 North Campbell Ave-
  nue
Tucson, AZ 85724

California

Charles R. Drew Univer-
  sity of Medicine and Sci-
  ence
12714 South Avalon Boule-
  vard, Suite 301
Los Angeles, CA 90061

City of Hope National Medical Center
Beckman Research Institute
1500 East Duarte Road
Duarte, CA 91010

Jonsson Comprehensive
Cancer Center
University of California Los
Angeles Medical Center
10-247 Factor Building
10833 LeConte Avenue
Los Angeles, CA 90024

The Kenneth Norris, Jr.,
Comprehensive Cancer
Center and
The Kenneth Norris, Jr.,
Hospital and Research Institute
University of Southern California
1441 Eastlake Avenue
Los Angeles, CA 90033-0804

Northern California Cancer
Program
1301 Shoreway Road
Belmont, CA 94002

University of California San
Diego Medical Center
Cancer Center
225 Dickinson Street
San Diego, CA 92103

Colorado

University of Colorado Cancer Center
4200 East Ninth Street,
Box B190
Denver, CO 80262

Connecticut

Yale University Comprehensive Cancer Center
333 Cedar Street
New Haven, CT 06510

District of Columbia

Howard University Comprehensive Cancer Center
2041 Georgia Avenue, NW
Washington, DC 20060

Vincent T. Lombardi Cancer
Research Center
Georgetown University Hospital
3800 Reservoir Road, NW
Washington, DC 20007

Florida

Sylvester Comprehensive
Cancer Center
University of Miami Medical
School
1475 Northwest Twelfth Avenue
Miami, FL 33136

Illinois

Illinois Cancer Council
36 South Wabash Avenue
Chicago, IL 60603

University of Chicago Cancer
Research Center
5841 South Maryland Avenue
Chicago, IL 60637

Iowa

University of Iowa Cancer
Center
650 Newton Road
Iowa City, IA 52242

Kentucky

Lucille Parker Markey Cancer Center
University of Kentucky Medical Center
800 Rose Street
Lexington, KY 40536-0093

Maryland

Johns Hopkins Oncology
Center
600 North Wolfe Street
Baltimore, MD 21205

Massachusetts

Beth Israel Hospital
330 Brookline Avenue
Boston, MA 02215

Dana-Farber Cancer Institute
44 Binney Street
Boston, MA 02115

Massachusetts General Hospital
32 Fruit Street
Boston, MA 02114

Michigan

Meyer L. Prentis Comprehensive Cancer Center of
Metropolitan Detroit
110 East Warren Avenue
Detroit, MI 48201

University of Michigan Cancer Center
101 Simpson Drive
Ann Arbor, MI 48109-0752

Minnesota

Mayo Comprehensive Cancer
Center
200 First Street, SW
Rochester, MN 55905

University of Minnesota
Hospitals and Clinics
420 Delaware Street, SE
Minneapolis, MN 55455

New Hampshire

Norris Cotton Cancer Center
Dartmouth-Hitchcock Medical Center
2 Maynard Street
Hanover, NH 03756

New York

Albert Einstein College of Medicine
1300 Morris Park Avenue
New York, NY 10461

Columbia University Cancer Center
Columbia-Presbyterian Medical Center
622 West 168th Street
New York, NY 10032

Memorial Sloan-Kettering Cancer Center
1275 York Avenue
New York, NY 10021

Mount Sinai School of Medicine
One Gustav L. Levy Place
New York, NY 10029

New York University Cancer Center
462 First Avenue
New York, NY 10016-9103

Roswell Park Memorial Institute
Elm and Carlton Streets
Buffalo, NY 14263

University of Rochester Cancer Center
Strong Memorial Hospital
601 Elmwood Avenue, Box 704
Rochester, NY 14642

North Carolina

Bowman Gray School of Medicine
Wake Forest University
300 South Hawthorne Road
Winston-Salem, NC 27103

Duke University Comprehensive Cancer Center
P.O. Box 3843
Durham, NC 27710

Lineberger Cancer Research Center
University of North Carolina School of Medicine
Chapel Hill, NC 27599

Oncology Research Center
North Carolina Baptist Hospital
300 South Hawthorne Road
Winston-Salem, NC 27103

Ohio

Case Western Reserve University
University Hospitals of
  Cleveland
Ireland Cancer Center
2074 Abinton Road
Cleveland, OH 44106

Ohio University Comprehensive Cancer Center
410 West Twelfth Avenue
Columbus, OH 43210

Pennsylvania

Fox-Chase Cancer Center
7701 Burholme Avenue
Philadelphia, PA 19111

Hahnemann University Hospital
Broad and Vine Streets
Philadelphia, PA 19102

Pittsburgh Cancer Institute
230 Lothrop Street
Pittsburgh, PA 15213-2592

University of Pennsylvania
  Cancer Center
Hospital of the University of
  Pennsylvania
3400 Spruce Street
Philadelphia, PA 19104

Rhode Island

Roger Williams General Hospital
825 Chalkstone Avenue
Providence, RI 02908

Tennessee

St. Jude Children's Research
  Hospital
332 North Lauderdale Street
Memphis, TN 38101

Texas

University of Texas M. D.
  Anderson Cancer Center
1515 Holcombe Boulevard
Houston, TX 77030

University of Texas Medical
  Branch Hospital
Eighth and Mechanic Streets
Galveston, TX 77550

Utah

Utah Regional Cancer Center
University of Utah Medical
  Center
50 North Medical Drive,
  Room 2C10
Salt Lake City, UT 84132

Vermont

Vermont Regional Cancer
  Center
University of Vermont
1 South Prospect Street
Burlington, VT 05401

Virginia

Massey Cancer Center
Medical College of
  Virginia
Virginia Commonwealth
  University
1200 East Broad Street
Richmond, VA 23298

University of Virginia Medi-
  cal Center
Primary Care Center, Room
  4520
Lee Street
Charlottesville, VA 22908

Washington

Fred Hutchinson Cancer Research Center
1124 Columbia Street
Seattle, WA 98104

Wisconsin

Wisconsin Clinical Cancer
  Center
600 Highland Avenue
Madison, WI 53792

Appendix D

Recommended Reading

Nancy Bruning, *Coping with Chemotherapy: How to Take Care of Yourself While Chemotherapy Takes Care of Cancer* (New York: The Dial Press, 1986).

Cancer Manual, eighth edition, published by American Cancer Society, 247 Commonwealth Avenue, Boston, MA 02116, 1990. Written for physicians, but contains much information that can be reviewed with an oncologist's help.

Chemotherapy and You: A Guide to Self-help During Treatment, published by and available at no charge through Office of Cancer Communications, National Cancer Institute, Building 31, Room 10A18, Bethesda, MD 20205, or call Cancer Information Service at 1-800-4-CANCER. Answers common questions, with an excellent description of usual side effects associated with each anticancer drug.

Cope magazine, P. O. Box 51722, Boulder, CO 80321-1722. A magazine devoted to cancer patients and their problems, with many helpful articles and hints.

Eating Hints: Recipes and Tips for Better Nutrition During Cancer Treatment, published by and available at no charge through Office of Cancer Communications, National Cancer Institute, Building 31, Room 10A18, Bethesda, MD 20205, or call Cancer Information Service at 1-800-4-CANCER. Good tips in regard to nausea, vomiting, mouth problems, constipation, heartburn, and other problems related to nutrition.

John Laszlo, *Understanding Cancer* (New York: Harper & Row, 1987). A good general overview of cancer and its treatment.

Mary-Ellen Siegel, *The Cancer Patient Handbook* (New York: Walker & Co., 1986).

Ruth Spear, "Coping with Chemotherapy," *New York Magazine*, November 24, 1986. A good discussion of chemotherapy side effects and practical hints on how to cope with them.

Taking Time, published by and available at no charge through Office of Cancer Communications, National Cancer Institute, Building 31, Room 10A18, Bethesda, MD 20205, or call Cancer Information Service at 1-800-4-CANCER. An excellent exploration of the emotional issues associated with cancer.

Informational newsletters concerning cancer in general and specific cancers, such as breast and prostate, are regularly listed in the *NCCS Networker*, published by National Coalition for Cancer Survivorship. 323 Eighth Street SW, Albuquerque, NM 87102.

Index